COMPACT *Research*

Genetic Testing

Current Issues

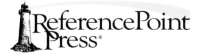

ReferencePoint Press®

San Diego, CA

Select* books in the Compact Research series include:

Current Issues

Animal Experimentation
Conflict in the Middle East
The Death Penalty
DNA Evidence and
    Investigation
Drugs and Sports
Gangs
Genetic Engineering
Genetic Testing
Gun Control

Immigration
Islam
National Security
Nuclear Weapons and
    Security
Obesity
Stem Cells
Teen Smoking
Terrorist Attacks
Video Games

Diseases and Disorders

ADHD
Alzheimer's Disease
Anorexia
Bipolar Disorders
HPV
Influenza

Mood Disorders
Post-Traumatic Stress
    Disorder
Self-Injury Disorder
Sexually Transmitted
    Diseases

Drugs

Antidepressants
Club Drugs
Cocaine and Crack
Heroin
Inhalants
Methamphetamine

Nicotine and Tobacco
Painkillers
Performance-Enhancing
    Drugs
Prescription Drugs
Steroids

Energy and the Environment

Biofuels
Coal Power
Deforestation
Energy Alternatives
Garbage and Recyling
Global Warming and
    Climate Change

Hydrogen Power
Nuclear Power
Solar Power
Toxic Waste
Wind Power
World Energy Crisis

*For a complete list of titles please visit www.referencepointpress.com.

Genetic Testing

Hal Marcovitz

Current Issues

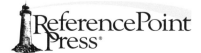

ReferencePoint
Press®

San Diego, CA

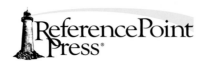

For more information, contact:
ReferencePoint Press, Inc.
PO Box 27779
San Diego, CA 92198
www.ReferencePointPress.com

Picture credits:
Cover: Dreamstime and iStockphoto.com
Maury Aaseng: 33–35, 48–49, 63–64, 77–79
AP Images: 13
Science Photo Library: 19

LIBRARY OF CONGRESS CATALOGING-IN-PUBLICATION DATA

Marcovitz, Hal.
  Genetic testing / by Hal Marcovitz.
    p. cm. — (Compact research)
  ISBN-13: 978-1-60152-115-6 (hardback)
  ISBN-10: 1-60152-115-4 (hardback)
  1. Human chromosome abnormalities—Diagnosis—Popular works. I. Title.
  RB155.6.M37   2011
  616'.042—dc22
                                                                    2010019581

Contents

Foreword

❝Where is the knowledge we have lost in information?❞

—T.S. Eliot, "The Rock."

As modern civilization continues to evolve, its ability to create, store, distribute, and access information expands exponentially. The explosion of information from all media continues to increase at a phenomenal rate. By 2020 some experts predict the worldwide information base will double every 73 days. While access to diverse sources of information and perspectives is paramount to any democratic society, information alone cannot help people gain knowledge and understanding. Information must be organized and presented clearly and succinctly in order to be understood. The challenge in the digital age becomes not the creation of information, but how best to sort, organize, enhance, and present information.

ReferencePoint Press developed the *Compact Research* series with this challenge of the information age in mind. More than any other subject area today, researching current issues can yield vast, diverse, and unqualified information that can be intimidating and overwhelming for even the most advanced and motivated researcher. The *Compact Research* series offers a compact, relevant, intelligent, and conveniently organized collection of information covering a variety of current topics ranging from illegal immigration and deforestation to diseases such as anorexia and meningitis.

The series focuses on three types of information: objective single-author narratives, opinion-based primary source quotations, and facts and statistics. The clearly written objective narratives provide context and reliable background information. Primary source quotes are carefully selected and cited, exposing the reader to differing points of view. And facts and statistics sections aid the reader in evaluating perspectives. Presenting these key types of information creates a richer, more balanced learning experience.

For better understanding and convenience, the series enhances information by organizing it into narrower topics and adding design features that make it easy for a reader to identify desired content. For example, in *Compact Research: Illegal Immigration*, a chapter covering the economic impact of illegal immigration has an objective narrative explaining the various ways the economy is impacted, a balanced section of numerous primary source quotes on the topic, followed by facts and full-color illustrations to encourage evaluation of contrasting perspectives.

The ancient Roman philosopher Lucius Annaeus Seneca wrote, "It is quality rather than quantity that matters." More than just a collection of content, the *Compact Research* series is simply committed to creating, finding, organizing, and presenting the most relevant and appropriate amount of information on a current topic in a user-friendly style that invites, intrigues, and fosters understanding.

Genetic Testing at a Glance

Genetic Testing Defined

Genetic testing is the medical procedure that examines variations in DNA to determine a patient's predisposition to develop diseases and disabilities.

Widespread Benefits

Genetic testing has revealed that some ethnic groups are predisposed to developing certain hereditary diseases. For instance, Jews of European descent can be carriers of Tay-Sachs disease and people of African descent can be carriers of sickle-cell anemia.

Uncovering Evidence of Disease

Genetic testing can alert people, sometimes decades in advance, of their likelihoods for developing breast and ovarian cancers, Huntington's disease, Alzheimer's disease, and other debilitating illnesses.

Nonmedical Applications

Genetic tests can help link criminals to crimes, help people trace their ancestries to different parts of the world, and even tell whether their children will be redheads.

Difficult Choices

Genetic tests often present people with difficult choices, such as whether to undergo major surgery to avoid severe illness or whether to terminate a pregnancy when tests show the baby will be born with debilitations.

Gender Selection

Genetic tests have long been able to predict the gender of a baby. When coupled with in vitro fertilization, couples can use genetic screening to select the gender of their child.

Privacy Issues

As genetic testing becomes more common, so do concerns about privacy. Civil libertarians worry that the FBI database of DNA profiles of convicted criminals and others is likely also to include the profiles of innocent people.

Legal Protections

Congress has outlawed the use of genetic information to deny people health insurance or employment opportunities, but doubts remain about how the results of genetic testing might be used.

Future Advancements

Genetic testing is expected to lead to the development of personalized medicine—the tailoring of drug therapies and treatments based on tests that reveal genetic mutations.

Overview

❝I don't come from a place of fear. I wanted to know so I could make plans. I have nieces, and wanted to inform my family.❞

—Sarah Thompson, a woman whose genetic test revealed that her breast cancer is not genetically related.

❝'Do I really want to know all about myself?' I wondered as I spat into a test tube to provide a DNA sample. What if I have a life sentence hanging over me?❞

—Cassandra Jardine, columnist for the *Daily Telegraph*, a newspaper based in London, England.

G enetic testing is the medical process to determine, in some cases several years beforehand, the likelihood that a patient will become afflicted with a disease or debilitation inherited from parents or other ancestors, or whether the patient is a carrier of genes that could afflict offspring with a disease. The test is performed through a biochemical analysis of the patient's genetic material—genes, chromosomes, proteins, and DNA.

The first genetic tests for disease were performed in the 1970s. For many years testing could provide evidence of only a handful of diseases and debilitations, but the list of conditions that can be identified through genetic screening now numbers more than 1,000. Experts believe the science will expand during the next few years, providing evidence of virtually all inherited diseases people are likely to face. Says Virginia Tech University professor Doris Teichler Zallen, an authority on genetic testing:

Genetic tests are designed to explore those tiny hereditary units—our genes—hidden away in each of the cells in our bodies. These tests probe the threadlike substance, DNA, of which genes are made, looking for any flaws. As we have come to know, even a small change in the genetic material can cause health problems. In some cases, these problems can show up right away; in other cases, they may make themselves known much later in life.[1]

For many people the science of genetic testing has raised troubling questions. Faced with overwhelming evidence that children would be born with disabilities, many couples have elected to abort pregnancies. For many adult patients, the truth about whether they face horrific diseases is not always made clear through genetic testing. They find themselves deciding whether to undergo life-changing surgeries for removal of organs even though, at the time of the test, there may be nothing wrong with them. And genetic testing has also prompted many people to fear that the results of their tests could be used as a tool of discrimination.

Race for a Cure

Jeff Carroll was 20 years old when his mother started showing symptoms of Huntington's disease. The disease, which is caused by mutated genes, usually manifests its symptoms in patients between the ages of 30 and 50. Early symptoms include forgetfulness, clumsiness, and mood swings. As Huntington's disease progresses, patients lose the ability to speak and walk; their limbs may thrash about in uncontrollable jerking movements. Although the disease itself is not fatal, complications such as pneumonia often end the lives of Huntington's patients 20 years or so after they begin showing symptoms.

Because of the mutated genes, the body's cells produce a certain protein that is harmful to the health of brain cells, which are known as neurons. Exposed to the protein, the neurons in Huntington's patients die much more quickly than in normal patients and are not replaced by healthy neurons.

For a patient to develop Huntington's disease, either of two genes can be mutated. When Carroll's mother was diagnosed with the disease, it meant that Carroll was likely to develop the disease himself. "I decided

> **For many years testing could provide evidence of only a handful of diseases and debilitations, but the list of conditions that can be identified through genetic screening now numbers more than 1,000.**

to get tested right away," Carroll says. "I had to know."[2] Soon, the genetic test revealed the truth: Carroll also tested positive for the mutated genes, meaning he would also develop Huntington's disease eventually.

In the years since his test, Carroll has forged a career as a neuroscience researcher at the University of British Columbia in Vancouver, Canada, and has joined a team searching for a cure for Huntington's disease. His research has focused on finding a drug that would help cells eliminate the protein that damages healthy neurons. Now in his thirties, Carroll knows he is in a race to find a cure because he could start manifesting the Huntington's symptoms at any time. "I'm doing what I can, and that's all I can do,"[3] says Carroll.

The Evolution of Gene Testing

In 1859 British naturalist Charles Darwin first suggested that many diseases run in families when he published his landmark book on evolution, *On the Origin of Species*. It would take nearly a century, though, before scientists understood how physical traits, including diseases, are passed on from generation to generation. In 1953 British scientists Francis Crick and James D. Watson discovered the structure of DNA, the molecule that contains voluminous amounts of information about the human body and how that information is passed on from parents to children.

Once scientists understood the nature of the DNA molecule, they were able to start developing ways to unearth its secrets. In 1961 medical researcher Robert Guthrie proposed that a simple blood test administered on newborns could determine whether children might develop phenylketonuria (PKU), which often causes mental retardation. In patients afflicted with PKU, the body is unable to break down phenylalanine, an amino acid found in food. An overabundance of phenylalanine in the body results in mental impairment.

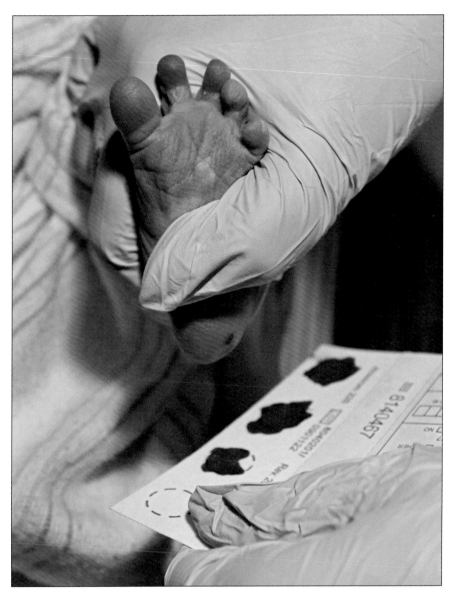

A day-old baby undergoes a simple heel prick to obtain blood for screening to detect the genetic disorder PKU and other conditions. Tests such as this allow for early detection and quick response, both of which can improve chances for a normal life.

Guthrie suspected that PKU was genetically related because his son as well as a niece were both mentally retarded, and both had tested positive for high levels of phenylalanine. By screening newborns, Guthrie said, parents could learn whether their children were afflicted with high levels of the amino acid and place them on diets low in phenylalanine. Meat, chicken, fish, nuts, and cheese all contain high levels of phenylalanine; by eliminating those foods, children born with PKU could go on to develop normal brains. Therefore the first genetic test did not examine genetic material but nevertheless showed how a genetically caused disease could be detected and avoided.

By the early 1970s widespread genetic testing had commenced for Tay-Sachs disease, a buildup of protein in the brain that affects mostly Jews of European descent, and sickle-cell anemia, which causes blockages of arteries and affects mostly people of African descent. Victims of Tay-Sachs usually die in early childhood, whereas sickle-cell anemia patients can be expected to live into adulthood but often die in their forties.

How Genes Are Tested

The DNA molecule resembles a twisted ladder—the double helix—that is composed of four base chemicals: adenine, guanine, cytosine, and thymine. In every DNA molecule these chemicals form bonds and pair up, creating some 3 billion combinations.

One person's DNA is not terribly different from the next person's. Of the 3 billion potential combinations of the four chemicals, there are only about 10 million places where the combinations differ from person to person. These variations are known as single nucleotide polymorphisms. They are responsible for the differences in people's hair and eye color, whether one person will be thin and wiry while another is short and stocky, and why one person will develop breast cancer while another person does not.

> " There are about 2 million proteins in the human body and, therefore, many opportunities for faulty proteins to cause mischief. "

The four DNA chemicals also switch on proteins, which are chemicals that carry out the functions of the body. There are about 2 million proteins in the human body and, therefore, many opportunities for faulty proteins to cause mischief.

Most cells in the body contain genes, which are tiny components that determine physical characteristics. Each human body is estimated to contain as many as 23,000 genes. The genes, which contain the body's DNA, are components of threadlike structures known as chromosomes. Each human cell normally contains 46 chromosomes in 23 matching pairs—1 chromosome in each pair is inherited from the mother and 1 from the father. (Twenty-two of the chromosomes are numbered; the twenty-third is labeled X or Y depending on gender. Females are XX, and males are XY). Each chromosome includes strings of genes.

> " **Genetic testing can uncover diseases that other tests have missed.** "

In most cases genetic screening is performed through an analysis of the genetic material contained in white blood cells or from the cells drawn from a small sample of tissue, often obtained from inside the cheek. In the case of a newborn, the blood sample is typically drawn from the baby's heel. In analyzing the blood or tissue sample, researchers look for a mutation of the gene that would lead to development of the disease in the patient. Through the study of patients who have developed particular diseases, researchers know how to recognize the variations on the DNA molecule known to cause many inherited diseases.

Beyond Medicine

DNA testing goes beyond medical applications. Police often use DNA evidence to link suspects to crimes. The first so-called DNA fingerprinting test was employed by police in 1984. By drawing a DNA sample from a suspect, a lab can match the sample to the DNA found in a smear of blood or strand of hair left at the scene of the crime.

DNA testing is also used to prove paternity. Errant fathers who balk at providing support for their children have been ordered by judges to provide financial support for their families after DNA tests prove they are, in fact, the biological fathers of the children.

DNA testing has also been used to provide answers to historical mysteries. In 2010 scientists announced the results of DNA tests on the 3,300-year-old remains of the Egyptian king Tutankhamen. The tests determined that the young King Tut, who died at the age of 19, suffered from malaria. Moreover, the DNA test of Tut's remains indicated that his parents were probably brother and sister.

How Beneficial Is Genetic Testing for Diseases?

Genetic testing can uncover diseases that other tests have missed. For example, so-called cancers of unknown primary origin are tumors that defy identification through ordinary tests, such as colonoscopies and mammograms. Genetic testing is effective in identifying these tumors and helping doctors tailor treatments to patients.

Jo Symons developed cancerous tumors in her neck, chest and lymph nodes. To treat Symons properly, doctors needed to know the origin of the tumors. She underwent a barrage of tests, but all the tests failed to detect the cause of the tumors. After several months of unsuccessful treatments, Symons underwent a genetic test that determined the cancer originated in her pancreas. Doctors immediately started treating her with drugs designed to combat cancer of the pancreas, but by then it was too late. The cancer had progressed too far, and she died shortly after the genetic test had helped doctors make the correct diagnosis.

> Among the most controversial aspects of genetic screening is when the test is performed on fetal cells, revealing that the child would be born with a disease or debilitation.

Her husband, John, is not sure whether a quicker diagnosis may have saved his wife's life, but he does encourage other patients with cancers of unknown primary origin to seek genetic testing. "It gave us comfort to identify where the cancer had come from," John Symons says. "It's very uncomfortable not knowing where a problem has arisen in your body."[4]

From Parents to Children

Many people find themselves unprepared for the harsh truths uncovered by their genetic tests. Feeling fine but aware that a disease runs in their family, they undergo testing and learn that they, too, may be facing cancer or another devastating illness in the future.

When the mother-in-law of novelist Susan Gregg Gilmore developed ovarian cancer, Gilmore started thinking about the illnesses that had stricken members of her own family. She decided to undergo a test that would determine whether she was genetically predisposed to developing cancer. The test showed mutations in Gilmore's BRCA genes, which are the genes that are responsible for the development of breast and ovarian cancer. People who test positive for the gene mutations have as much as a 60 percent chance of developing cancer. In 2007 Gilmore underwent surgery to have her healthy ovaries removed.

> **The case of pro basketball player Eddy Curry serves as an example of somebody who faced discrimination based on the fear of what a genetic test might show.**

Now, Gilmore must also live with the knowledge that her daughter, Claudia, may have inherited the same gene mutation. "As a parent, you know bad things are going to happen to your kids," says Gilmore. "But it's a very different feeling when you are the ones handing them the muck."[5]

How Do Genetic Tests Influence Family Planning?

Among the most controversial aspects of genetic screening is when the test is performed on fetal cells, revealing that the child would be born with a disease or debilitation. Parents who learn the truth about what awaits their offspring find themselves facing the question of whether to terminate the pregnancies. As such, the science of genetic testing has been placed squarely at the center of the abortion debate in America.

Many opponents of abortion remain steadfast in their opposition to the procedure, even if the test shows the child would be born with a painful disease or severe mental impairment. Says a statement by the United States Conference of Catholic Bishops:

> Knowledge of genetic defects responsible for disease allows science to conduct a directed search for cures; screens can then reveal who needs treatment. . . . Unfortunately, such information can also tempt people toward decisions

the Church recognizes as objectively wrong. . . . Abortion is never a morally acceptable response. Rather, it is a raw and lethal assertion of one human being's power over another.[6]

Zallen, who supports abortion rights, counters that abortion should remain an option for parents who learn their child will be born with a horrific disease or debilitation. She says:

People who have decided to end a much-wanted pregnancy often feel they have no other option. This may be because they lack the emotional or financial resources to care for a child born with a serious illness, or that they are already physically drained by caring for another child with the same disorder, or because they are coping with any number of distressing life circumstances. Even people who are staunchly anti-abortion in theory have found themselves making the painful choice to end a pregnancy based on genetic test results.[7]

Will Genetic Testing Lead to Discrimination?

People who learn they are facing diseases later in life often harbor fears about discrimination. Would a person be fired if the employer learns that the person is likely to develop cancer? Would an insurance company, knowing it may be hit with massive medical bills, kick an otherwise healthy patient off an insurance plan out of fear that in the near future the patient will develop a disease that would cost hundreds of thousands of dollars to treat?

Lawmakers have taken steps to ensure that people do not face loss of their health insurance or jobs based on genetic evidence, but doubts remain. Indeed, the case of pro basketball player Eddy Curry serves as an example of somebody who faced discrimination based on the fear of what a genetic test might show.

In 2005 Curry, a player for the Chicago Bulls, exhibited symptoms of an irregular heartbeat. Curry was administered a battery of tests and cleared to play, but Bulls management suspected Curry may suffer from the potentially fatal heart disease known as hypertrophic cardiomyopa-

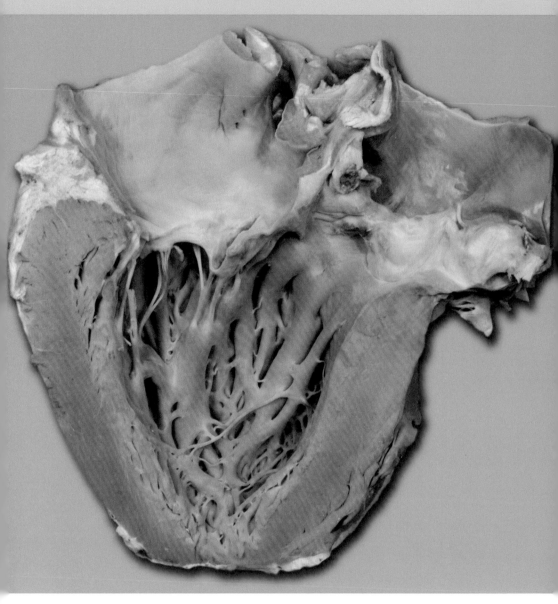

When the Chicago Bulls ordered player Eddy Curry to undergo genetic testing for hypertrophic cardiomyopathy, Curry refused. This condition involves the thickening of the heart muscle and is a major cause of death in young athletes who seem healthy but die during heavy exercise. Curry feared the team would use the results against him. Pictured here is a heart afflicted by this condition.

thy. This condition results when the heart muscle thickens. Because of the thickening, the heart has to work harder to pump blood. The first

> **Now that the human genome has been mapped, genetic screening is expected to progress quickly during the next few years, uncovering new truths about how diseases develop in the body.**

symptom of hypertrophic cardiomyopathy among many young patients is sudden collapse and possible death caused by abnormal heart rhythms. Hypertrophic cardiomyopathy is a major cause of death in young athletes who seem completely healthy but die during heavy exercise. Bulls management wanted Curry to undergo genetic testing to find out if he suffered from this condition. The team may have been concerned about more than just the player's health—it was about to offer Curry a $5 million contract. "If we as an organization don't explore everything that's available, then we're being negligent," insisted Bulls general manager John Paxson. "All we've asked, all along . . . is that he just go a little bit further in terms of evaluation."[8]

Curry refused to take the test. His attorney predicted that the Bulls would set a dangerous precedent by showing that employers could fire workers based on the outcome of their DNA tests. Curry's lawyer, Alan Milstein, said:

> Think about what's at stake here. As far as DNA testing, we're just at the beginning of that universe. Pretty soon, though, we'll know whether someone is predisposed to cancer, alcoholism, obesity, baldness and who knows what else. Hand that information to an employer and imagine the implications. If the NBA were to get away with it, what about everyone else in the country looking for a job?[9]

When Curry refused to take the test, the Bulls traded him to the New York Knicks. Since the trade, Curry has continued his career in New York and appears by all accounts to be healthy.

Although genetic testing was first employed decades ago, the science took tremendous steps forward in 2003 with the completion of the Human Genome Project, which mapped every gene in the human body.

The project was conducted in separate private and government-funded facilities. *Genome* is a term applied to the entire genetic composition of an organism. Therefore, by mapping the human genome—identifying every gene in the body and its functions—the Human Genome Project has provided physicians with an overall picture of how genes interact, evolve, and mutate.

Now that the human genome has been mapped, genetic screening is expected to progress quickly during the next few years, uncovering new truths about how diseases develop in the body. Says Zallen, "The more we know about the human gene map, the easier it is to find a target gene."[10]

The Science Advances

Genetic testing is heading into directions that were probably not envisioned by scientists when the mysteries of DNA were first unraveled decades ago. Some of those directions promise to enhance the delivery of health care. For example, doctors have started prescribing certain specific medications to patients whose tests indicate how their individual genetic makeup affects the absorption of the drugs into their bodies.

While most people involved with the delivery of health care endorse such steps forward, many medical experts are not as sure about some of the other advances that have been attributed to genetic testing. Already, it is possible to learn through genetic testing the gender of babies before they are born. In recent years the science has advanced even further, making it possible in some cases actually to select the gender of children. Critics question whether doctors step over the line when they enable parents to select the gender of their babies. Says University of Chicago bioethicist Leon Kass, "Even though some of us have strong differences of opinion on some issues, all of us have a stake in keeping human reproduction human."[11]

Despite such fears expressed by Kass and other critics, gender selection remains an option for some parents. In the future it is likely that many more people will find themselves knowing and even picking the gender of their children before birth as well as learning the many other new truths about themselves and their families that will be made available through genetic testing.

How Beneficial Is Genetic Testing for Diseases?

❝If they waited for symptoms to develop, they probably would have suffered the same fate as their siblings—which would be to die of a very aggressive stomach cancer.❞

—Laurence McCahill, a California cancer surgeon commenting on cases in which patients had their stomachs removed after genetic tests indicated their chances of developing cancer.

❝Most carrier tests are designed to look for the common mutations. If you are told you don't have any of the common mutations, it substantially reduces your risk of being a carrier, but it doesn't eliminate the risk completely.❞

—Doris Teichler Zallen, a professor at Virginia Tech University and authority on genetic testing.

Disease with Family Connections

Some diseases run in families. Traits that cause diseases are buried in people's DNA and passed down from generation to generation. Every person inherits two copies of every gene—one from each parent. Mutations of these genes can cause diseases on their own or work in concert with other genes to cause mischief.

Some diseases are inherited through dominant genes. A dominant gene can determine a specific trait or condition on its own. Huntington's disease is caused by a dominant gene; a person who inherits a single copy of the flawed gene that causes the disease has a 50 percent chance of developing the disease. A person who inherits copies of the gene from both parents would almost surely develop Huntington's.

Other diseases are caused by recessive genes. In such cases diseases will not develop unless copies of the gene mutation are inherited from both parents. Cystic fibrosis, a potentially fatal condition that causes thick, sticky mucus to build up in the lungs, is caused by recessive genes. A person who inherits copies of the gene from both parents is likely to develop cystic fibrosis. On the other hand, a person who inherits one copy of the gene from one parent will not develop the disease. But this person is still a carrier and may pass the gene on to a child. The child's chances of developing cystic fibrosis will depend on whether the other parent is also a carrier.

> " Genetic tests are unlike other forms of medical testing because in many cases the patient feels fine and is being tested for an illness that may not show symptoms for decades. "

Many other diseases stem from multigenic conditions, meaning they are caused by multiple genes influencing one another. In addition, environmental factors—such as smoking and diet—also influence genes and may spark them into mutating.

Mental Anguish

In an ordinary medical test, the patient may have gone to the doctor because he or she may feel pain or other symptoms and suspects an illness may be the cause. The patient may be somewhat mentally prepared for the bad news. However, genetic tests are unlike other forms of medical testing because in many cases the patient feels fine and is being tested for an illness that may not show symptoms for decades. Doctors and genetic counselors report that many people who undergo genetic testing suffer from severe mental anguish as they wait for the results and further anguish when they ultimately learn they have tested positive for a flawed gene that might cause a future illness.

Karen Belz, an English teacher from Boston, Massachusetts, experienced mental anguish while waiting for her test results. Belz's mother, Eva, died from breast cancer. When Belz's older sister, Ruth, developed a malignant tumor in one breast, Belz decided to undergo testing for mutations in the BRCA1 and BRCA2 genes, which are the two genes responsible for causing breast and ovarian cancer. "I can't continue in this limbo," she said. "I have to know."[12]

Belz underwent the testing at Beth Israel Deaconess Medical Center near Boston. Because of the mental trauma suffered by patients, the hospital has established a procedure that lets the patient pick the time to be told the results. Patients can delay the news indefinitely or elect not to be told at all if they decide, during the waiting period, that they are not emotionally capable of learning the news.

Belz waited five weeks. The test revealed that she carries the same genetic mutations that afflicted her mother and sister. Rather than wait for what she believed would be the inevitable arrival of cancer, Belz elected to have surgery to remove her breasts and ovaries.

The anguish of learning about the existence of a faulty gene can be extreme, especially when that gene may lead to an illness for which there is no cure. Faced with such a cold reality, these patients can take steps that would help minimize the impact of the disease on their families. Many carriers organize their financial affairs so resources are available to care for them when they are no longer able to care for themselves. Many carriers forgo having children rather than take the chance of passing mutated genes on to their offspring. Says a statement by the New York–based Hereditary Disease Foundation, "Those who choose to be tested usually do so in order to be able to make informed plans for the future regarding marriage, reproduction, career, finances and so on. Others may simply crave relief from the anguish of being 'at risk.' For them, knowing, whatever the outcome, is better than not knowing."[13]

Risk-Reduction Surgery

Many people who receive positive tests for cancer elect to undergo surgeries even though they have not yet developed symptoms. The family of Natasha Benn was afflicted with stomach cancer—several relatives died from the disease. When her sister was diagnosed with a malignant tumor in her stomach, Benn underwent genetic testing that revealed, as she fully expected, that she carried the same gene mutation that had taken the lives of family members. Doctors told her that she had an 80 percent chance of developing stomach cancer. Benn elected to have her stomach removed. Said Benn, of Victoria, Canada, "It was something I had to do for myself and my family, so they didn't have to worry about me."[14]

Benn, as well as Karen Belz, underwent what is known as risk-reduction surgery. They had parts of their bodies removed before those organs were afflicted with cancerous tumors. In addition to breasts, ovaries, and stomachs, surgeons have removed colons, thyroid glands, and uteruses.

> **They had parts of their bodies removed before those organs were afflicted with cancerous tumors.**

People can live without their stomachs. Patients are advised to eat small portions of food, which can be digested by the small intestine. After Benn underwent the surgery, four other members of her family were genetically screened, and all four had their stomachs removed as well. In all cases, examinations of their stomach tissue showed precancerous conditions, meaning that cancer was likely to develop.

Inconclusive Results

Even with genetic testing becoming more sophisticated, experts concede that the test results can be inconclusive. A genetic test may show a mutated gene—but the test may not indicate the degree to which the gene has mutated or that the mutation is likely to cause disease. "Not all mutations are equal," says Doris Teichler Zallen, "and the risk figure you will be given is most likely going to be a range, say 50–85 percent by the age of 70. Admittedly, we are just at the beginning of the era of genetic medicine, and medical experience with specific gene mutations is still limited."[15]

Inconclusive results are common in genetic screening for breast and ovarian cancers. The National Cancer Institute points out that a negative test result is no guarantee that a patient with a family history of breast cancer will avoid the disease. "In cases in which a family has a history of breast or ovarian cancer and no known mutation in BRCA1 or BRCA2 has been previously identified, a negative test result is not informative," concludes an institute publication. "It is possible for people to have a mutation in a gene other than BRCA1 or BRCA2 that increases their cancer risk but is not detectable by the tests used."[16]

These type of cases are regarded as ambiguous. According to the National Cancer Institute, 10 percent of women whose tests show they do not carry mutations of the BRCA1 and BRCA2 genes are told that their results are ambiguous and that they still may develop genetically based breast or ovarian cancers.

Testing After the Illness Is Discovered

Many doctors advocate genetic testing for patients even after they have been diagnosed with cancer or other illnesses. The reason? If doctors know there is a genetic component to the illness, the treatment and drug therapy may be altered.

Cancers caused through genetic mutations are often much more aggressive than cancers attributed to environmental factors, such as diet or exposure to harmful chemicals. Some cancer patients believe that if they had known there was a genetic element to their illnesses, they would have undergone more radical surgeries or stronger chemotherapy and radiation treatments. After undergoing the lesser treatments, they are faced with the realization that their cancers may recur. "For many people . . . their genetic testing came too late, well after the treatment decisions had been made,"[17] says Zallen.

> **Cancers caused through genetic mutations are often much more aggressive than cancers attributed to environmental factors, such as diet or exposure to harmful chemicals.**

In Heather Bakstad's case, she was tested after her diagnosis and learned that her disease is not genetically related. The Seattle, Washington, real estate agent feels she has a much better chance of recovery now that she knows there is not a genetic component to her cancer. Bakstad says she was prepared to undergo a double mastectomy—a procedure in which both breasts are removed. With the diagnosis showing the cancer was not genetically related, doctors concluded the operation was unnecessary. "I would have done a double mastectomy for sure," she says. "It does mean I have a better outcome and prognosis because the test was negative."[18]

Solving Medical Mysteries

Genetic testing has unearthed causes for diseases that have defied explanation for decades. In 2008 genetic tests revealed that children who have a missing or duplicated series of chromosomes are 100 times more likely than other children to develop autism, a neural disorder that often slows a child's abilities to communicate or interact with others.

Six out of every 1,000 American children are born with autism. Symptoms of autism usually surface by the time a child reaches the age of three. But doctors believe that if a baby tests positive for autism, the parents can place the child in a therapeutic program at an earlier age, which could enhance the child's chances of developing normally.

"When parents have a child diagnosed with an autism spectrum disorder, one of the first questions they often ask is, 'How did this happen?'" says Robert Marion, a pediatric geneticist at Children's Hospital at Montefiore Medical Center in New York City. "In the vast majority of cases, we believe there is at least a genetic predisposition to autism."[19]

> " In 2007 genetic tests revealed that as many as half of people of European descent carry a gene mutation that increases the risk of heart disease. "

Millions May Potentially Benefit from Discoveries

The discoveries of the genetic components of Tay-Sachs and sickle-cell anemia show how entire ethnic groups can be affected by genetic testing. In 2007 genetic tests revealed that as many as half of people of European descent carry a gene mutation that increases the risk of heart disease.

The genetic mutation is so common that tests have indicated that at least 50 percent of people of European descent carry 1 copy of the flawed gene, and 20 percent carry 2 copies. This means millions of people who

> **Physicians and social scientists caution that even people with 'good genes' are susceptible to disease due to environmental factors, poor diets, smoking, and similar abuses.**

live in Europe as well as North America and other places where Europeans have migrated are likely to be afflicted with genetic predispositions that cause heart disease. The scientists who discovered the mutation hope to be able to develop tests that will tell individuals whether they are carriers. These individuals can then take steps to lower their blood pressure or change their diets to reduce the level of artery-clogging cholesterol in their bodies. Says Thomas Hughes, head of diabetes research for the drug company Novartis, "Things that were deeply buried in our [genes] . . . start to shine when you pool them with larger and larger populations."[20]

Genes Do Not Tell the Whole Story

Physicians and social scientists caution that even people with "good genes" are susceptible to disease due to environmental factors, poor diets, smoking, and similar abuses. They worry that people may adopt a false sense of security if they test negative for certain disease-causing genes. "It's no wonder that we have come to regard ourselves as exclusively defined by our genes,"[21] says Zallen. She worries that people who believe their genes are healthy may pay less attention to other factors that could cause disease, such as lifestyle choices, infectious diseases, and exposure to toxins and workplace chemicals.

Still, it is likely that as testing becomes more widespread, more people will make use of the information provided by their genes. They may find it necessary to change their diets or make other alterations to their lifestyles, such as finding jobs that do not place them in contact with chemicals that could work in concert with their mutated genes, further enhancing their chances of getting ill. Many individuals may elect to undergo removal of their breasts, ovaries, or other parts of their bodies, finding that the surgeries are a better alternative than waiting for cancer to arrive.

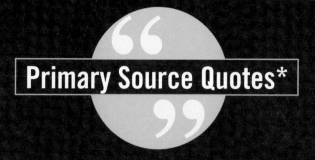

Primary Source Quotes*

How Beneficial Is Genetic Testing for Diseases?

66Genetic tests can offer glimpses into—or predictions about—the future. Unlike other types of tests that are snapshots of a person's health at the moment of testing, a genetic test can alert people who are perfectly healthy right now that they may be at significant risk for having a particular disorder in the years or decades ahead.99

—Doris Teichler Zallen, *To Test or Not to Test.* New Brunswick, NJ: Rutgers University Press, 2008.

Zallen is a professor of science and technology in society at Virginia Tech University.

66I can recall many professional lectures I attended which indicted that 'genetic knowledge was coming at us like a freight train.' Well, if that's true, then the freight train is moving faster than ever.99

—Carrie A. Zabel, Welcome to the Genetics Blog, Mayo Clinic, October 4, 2008. www.mayoclinic.com.

Zabel is the genetic test counselor at the Mayo Clinic, the medical center in Rochester, Minnesota, regarded as one of the top research-oriented hospitals in America.

* Editor's Note: While the definition of a primary source can be narrowly or broadly defined, for the purposes of Compact Research, a primary source consists of: 1) results of original research presented by an organization or researcher; 2) eyewitness accounts of events, personal experience, or work experience; 3) first-person editorials offering pundits' opinions; 4) government officials presenting political plans and/or policies; 5) representatives of organizations presenting testimony or policy.

Primary Source Quotes

❝In some cases, a negative result might not give any useful information. This type of result is called uninformative, indeterminate, inconclusive, or ambiguous. Uninformative test results sometimes occur because everyone has common, natural variations of their DNA, called polymorphisms, that do not affect health.❞

—Lister Hill National Center for Biomedical Communications, *Genetics Home Reference.* Bethesda, MD: U.S. National Library of Medicine/LHNCBC, 2009.

Lister Hill National Center for Biomedical Communications is the research division of the U.S. National Library of Medicine, an agency of the National Institutes of Health.

❝My cousin Sarah, six years younger than I am, found a lump while breast-feeding her new daughter. It was an aggressive cancer, and the prognosis was not great. Her doctors had also identified a faulty gene—BRCA2—which meant that anyone in Sarah's family, including third-degree relatives like me, was also at risk.❞

—Dominique Jackson, "One Woman's Journey: Taking the Risk of Breast Cancer Seriously," *Seattle Post-Intelligencer,* April 9, 2010.

Jackson is a staff writer for *Marie Claire* magazine.

❝On the downside, I have a slightly raised risk of breast cancer, 7.2 percent rather than 6.7 percent for women in their fifties. My profile couldn't tell me whether this risk is associated with the presence of the genes BRCA1 and BRCA2 because it is mutations in those genes rather than the genes themselves that are at high risk.❞

—Cassandra Jardine, "A Dip in the Gene Pool Reveals What I'm Made Of," *Daily Telegraph,* June 2, 2008.

Jardine is a columnist for the *Daily Telegraph,* a newspaper based in London, England.

66A group of researchers at Georgetown Medical Center asked relatives of carriers of BRCA mutations whether they wanted to know their own status. A majority agreed—but among the minority who did not, depression frequently took hold.99

—Masha Gessen, *Blood Matters: From Inherited Illness to Designer Babies, How the World and I Found Ourselves in the Future of the Gene*. New York: Harcourt, 2008.

Gessen, a Russian-born journalist, underwent a double mastectomy after learning she carries mutations of the genes that cause breast cancer.

66The emotional hell caused by genetic testing is amazing. Cancer therapy providers should do a better job of preparing the patient for this event in their lives.99

—Mark Sanford, *Cancer's Spouse*. Morrisville, NC: Lulu, 2007.

Sanford's wife, Glenna, was diagnosed with breast cancer; after her diagnosis, Glenna underwent a genetic test that indicated she carried the BRCA gene mutation. As a result of her diagnosis, Glenna agreed to undergo surgical removal of her uterus, which could also have developed cancer due to the BRCA gene mutation.

66My doctor cautioned me not to become anxious about the test results. She said that nothing had changed: I had always had the genetic mutation, and knowing about it did not mean I had cancer. But still, it wasn't good news.99

—Michelle Meklir McBride, "BRCA Journal: The Journey of a New Mom," *SU2C*, 2009. http://su2c.standup2cancer.org.

McBride is an attorney and advocate for cancer patients in Chicago, Illinois.

Facts and Illustrations

How Beneficial Is Genetic Testing for Diseases?

- In America breast cancer strikes about **1 in 8 women**, but only 1 in 500 people—men and women—carry mutations of the BRCA genes.

- Women who carry mutated BRCA genes have an **80 percent** chance of developing breast cancer and a **60 percent** chance of developing ovarian cancer in their lifetimes. Mothers who carry the mutated genes have a **50 percent** chance of passing them on to their children.

- A 2009 study by the National Cancer Institute reported that DNA testing is **25 percent** more effective in detecting cervical cancer than the Pap smear, which is an analysis of cells withdrawn from the cervix.

- According to Harvard University Medical School, the results of most genetic tests are available from **two to six weeks** after they are administered.

- A study conducted in Israel found that only **half the participants** said they would want to know results of genetic screening for Huntington's disease; when asked about genetic screening for cancer, more than **80 percent** said they would want to know the results.

- Medical researchers have identified four genes responsible for sparking Alzheimer's disease; as many as **75 percent** of people who carry the gene mutations for Alzheimer's will develop the disease by the age of 85.

Risk-Reduction Surgery Helps Prevent Breast Cancer

Genetic testing can identify women who are more likely to develop certain types of breast cancer, giving them the option of undergoing potentially life-saving risk-reduction surgery. A study published in the *Journal of Clinical Oncology* shows that risk-reduction surgery helps prevent the types of breast cancer that occur in women who test positive for mutations in the BRCA1 and BRCA2 genes. In that study, 19 women (about 6 percent) who underwent preventative mastectomies eventually developed cancers, while 28 (nearly 10 percent) of those who chose not to undergo preventative surgery developed breast cancer.

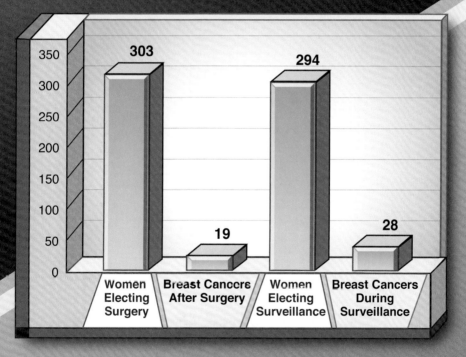

Note: Physicians monitored the patients for 23 months.

Source: Noah D. Kauff et al., "Risk-Reducing Salpingo-Oophorectomy for the Prevention of BRCA1- and BRCA2-Associated Breast and Gynecological Cancer: A Multicenter, Prospective Study," *Journal of Clinical Oncology*, March 10, 2008, p. 1,331. http://jco.ascopubs.org.

- Medical researchers have discovered more than **400 gene mutations** responsible for triggering cystic fibrosis.

Public Divided on Genetic Testing

Should genetic testing be done for a disease when no treatment for that disease exists? Experts in genetic testing and medical ethics disagree on this question. A national poll commissioned by C.S. Mott Children's Hospital of the University of Michigan shows that members of the public are also divided on this topic.

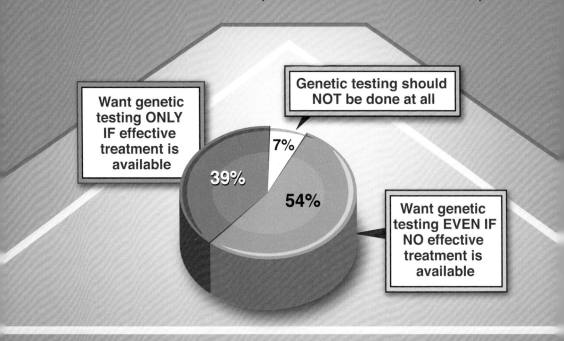

Want genetic testing ONLY IF effective treatment is available

Genetic testing should NOT be done at all

7%

39%

54%

Want genetic testing EVEN IF NO effective treatment is available

Source: C.S. Mott Children's Hospital National Poll on Children's Health, "Genetic Testing and DNA Biobanks—For Whom and When?" June 20, 2007. www.med.umich.edu.

- Amyotrophic lateral sclerosis (ALS), also known as Lou Gehrig's disease because it afflicted New York Yankee great Lou Gehrig, is sparked by the mutation in a single gene; about **10 percent** of ALS patients test positive for the gene mutation.

- Colon cancer afflicts about **6 percent** of the American adult population; as many as **80 percent** of people who carry the gene mutation that sparks colon cancer can expect to develop the disease.

Odds of Carrying a Faulty Gene

The genes for hereditary diseases such as sickle-cell anemia, cystic fibrosis, and the blood disorder beta-thalassemia occur more often in some racial and ethnic groups than others. Genetic testing can determine whether a person carries one of these genes. Hereditary diseases such as these usually occur when a child inherits the faulty gene from both parents.

Carrier frequency by population and condition

	Cystic fibrosis	Beta-thalassemia	Sickle cell
African American	1 in 65	1 in 75	1 in 12
Ashkenazi Jews	1 in 26–29		
European American	1 in 25–29		
Hispanic	1 in 46	1 in 30–50	
Mediterranean	1 in 29	1 in 25	1 in 40

Note: Disease genes are less common in some populations.

Source: *Washington Post*, "Odds of Carrying a Problem Gene," February 18, 2010. www.washingtonpost.com.

How Does Genetic Testing Influence Family Planning?

66There are many couples who do not want to have a baby with Down syndrome. They don't have the resources, don't have the emotional stamina, don't have the family support. We are recommending this testing be offered so that parents have a choice.99

—Deborah A. Driscoll, chief of obstetrics at the Hospital of the University of Pennsylvania.

66Today, nine out of 10 American women who are told they have a child with Down syndrome choose to abort. I think it's fair to say that if some of these potential parents had a glimpse of the other side they might have made a different decision.99

—Lon Jacobs, a New York City attorney and father of a daughter with Down syndrome.

Genetic Testing in the Womb

Greg and Tierney Fairchild first learned their baby would be born with a birth defect through an ultrasound, a routine procedure that uses sound waves to create images of the fetus in the womb. The ultrasound revealed their baby's heart had developed a hole between two chambers. Their physician feared further complications. The doctor knew that the condition, known as an endocardial cushion defect, could be an indication of a chromosomal disorder and that 60 percent of fetuses that develop the defect are born with a mentally and physically debilitating condition known as Down syndrome.

To learn the truth, Tierney Fairchild underwent a genetic test. For many years, the test has been performed through an amniocentesis—a procedure in which doctors insert a needle into the mother's abdomen, withdrawing about 1 ounce (30ml) of amniotic fluid. The fluid surrounds the fetus in the womb and is rich in fetal cells, which means it contains the baby's DNA. After the fluid is withdrawn, a genetic analysis can determine mutations that trigger inherited diseases.

Most physicians recommend the test if the patient has a family history of inherited diseases, if another test suggests a problem pregnancy, or if the mother is over 35. The age of the mother is often a factor in Down syndrome births. The odds of having a child with Down syndrome at age 40 is about 1 in 100. At age 35, the odds are about 1 in 350. The odds of having a child with Down syndrome at age 20 is about 1 in 2,000. It is unclear why women 35 and older are more likely to give birth to Down syndrome babies; some researchers suggest DNA breaks down in the eggs of older women.

Amniocentesis is a form of what is known as prenatal DNA testing. These tests have sparked debate because parents who receive the news that their children would be born with incurable diseases have the option of terminating the pregnancies. In actuality, most do: As many as 93 percent of women who learn through genetic testing that their babies will be born with Down syndrome elect to terminate their pregnancies, according to the National Institutes of Health.

As for the Fairchilds, they elected to go through with the pregnancy. Said Greg Fairchild, "We've made a decision based on our belief that whatever the range of problems are, between us and our family we are going to be able to get through it."[22]

The Ethics of Prenatal Testing

Critics suggest there is little difference between prenatal testing and old-fashioned eugenics, which proposed that if ill or mentally infirm people were barred from reproducing, the genetic pool of humanity would improve. The notion was first suggested by Francis Galton, a cousin of Charles Darwin. Galton believed that evolution could be given a nudge by ensuring high achievers married others of their class, thus producing offspring of superior abilities.

Eugenics was more than an intellectual movement. In 1927 the U.S. Supreme Court heard a case involving the involuntary sterilization of a mentally retarded woman. The woman, Carrie Buck, was born to a mentally retarded mother and had a daughter who was believed to be intellectually impaired as well. When the Virginia state institution where Buck lived proposed sterilizing her, civil libertarians sued to stop the procedure. Ultimately, the nation's highest court ruled against Buck. "Three generations of imbeciles are enough,"[23] wrote Justice Oliver Wendell Holmes Jr. Soon after the ruling, Buck was sterilized.

> " Critics suggest there is little difference between prenatal testing and old-fashioned eugenics. "

Eugenics lost favor after World War II as the horrific genetic experiments of the Nazi regime were revealed. (Nazi doctors were found to have experimented on concentration camp inmates, attempting, for example, to change the color of their eyes. In other bizarre and inhuman experiments, thousands of twins were murdered and their bodies dissected to discover genetic links.) Today doctors, parents, and bioethicists wrestle with such issues as whether the mother or the fetus is the patient, whether the fetus has legal rights, and whether the presence of a faulty gene justifies abortion.

The Case for Compassionate Abortion

Advocates for prenatal testing argue that women who opt for abortions after learning their children may be born with incurable diseases are choosing to undergo "compassionate abortions." They suggest these abortions free the children from a lifetime of pain and suffering. Such abortions, they say, also free families from the burdens of caring for these children, many of whom may require round-the-clock custodial care. "If amniocentesis reduced the number of mothers caring for profoundly disabled children, then the abortions that would result would be compassionate ones, entirely justified as a benefit to families,"[24] contends Ruth

Schwartz Cowan, a sociology professor at the University of Pennsylvania in Philadelphia.

Opponents counter that parents have an obligation to raise their children—regardless of their disabilities. "While the prospect of giving birth to a child who will have severe birth defects is a difficult challenge, do we as humans have the right to end the life of another simply because we feel their quality of life or personal worth is inferior to others?"[25] asks William McKeever, a Mormon leader and abortion opponent.

McKeever also points out that genetic tests are occasionally wrong. Such arguments were fueled in 2010 when health officials in Scotland disclosed the case of a man they identified as "Mr. C"—the individual preferred to remain anonymous—who tested positive in 1989 for the gene mutation that causes Huntington's disease. Believing he had the disease—and that he would pass the gene mutation on to his children and grandchildren—the man's wife and daughter terminated their pregnancies. Moreover, Mr. C lived in fear for the next two decades, waiting for the debilitating symptoms to take over his body.

> " A few weeks after her amniocentesis, the doctor called with the news: Her baby would be afflicted with Down syndrome. "

They never did. Finally, the man was retested. The new test showed that he did not carry the mutated gene, and therefore his wife and daughter had needlessly terminated their pregnancies.

A More Difficult Life

Julia Langdon waited until she was 36 before starting a family. Because she was over 35, Langdon elected to undergo genetic testing. A few weeks after her amniocentesis, the doctor called with the news: Her baby would be afflicted with Down syndrome. After hearing the doctor's report, Langdon had an abortion.

Down syndrome is caused by a chromosomal imbalance—babies are born with 47 chromosomes rather than the normal 46. Children born with Down syndrome face a lifetime of physical and cognitive impairments; most suffer moderate mental retardation, fail to grow normal physical features, and die in their forties.

Langdon looked at those obstacles and decided to terminate her pregnancy. "For me, the decision . . . was not about the rights and wrongs of abortion," says Langdon. "It was only about not wishing to bring a disabled child into the world, a child whose life would be more difficult."[26]

Living on Their Own

Abortion opponents and others argue that even Down syndrome children deserve a chance at life. Many parents of Down syndrome children have seen how their sons and daughters embrace life. Certainly, anybody who has attended a Special Olympics event has seen the intensity with which many of the young athletes pursue their competitions.

Nicole Springer, a Texas woman, elected to have her child even though prenatal testing indicated her daughter, Katarina, would be born with Down syndrome. "I can't imagine what my life would have been like if I'd chosen to terminate, if I didn't see that smile,"[27] Springer says of her daughter.

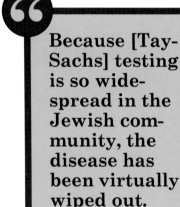

" Because [Tay-Sachs] testing is so widespread in the Jewish community, the disease has been virtually wiped out. "

Parents of Down syndrome children point out that society has become more accepting of them—decades ago, it was not unusual for states to institutionalize people with Down syndrome. Now it is more common for adult Down syndrome patients to hold jobs and live in group homes or other independent situations where they take care of their own needs, often with the assistance of visiting social workers. "I think people had the idea they were more trouble and more limited than they are,"[28] says Cynthia Coon, whose son Matthew, a Down syndrome patient, graduated from high school and has worked most of his adult life.

How Prenatal Testing Has Wiped Out Tay-Sachs

Children born with Tay-Sachs suffer from blindness, severe weakness, and an inability to react to stimuli. Few Tay-Sachs children live beyond the age of eight. The disease is triggered by a gene mutation located on the fifteenth chromosome and found mostly in the population of Jews of European descent, known as Ashkenazi Jews.

The first widespread genetic screenings for the disease were performed in 1970. To organize a national screening program, many influential Jewish leaders sponsored tests in synagogues and Jewish community centers. At the time testing commenced, between 50 and 60 Tay-Sachs babies were born in America each year. Because testing is so widespread in the Jewish community, the disease has been virtually wiped out. In 2003 no Ashkenazi Jewish child was born with Tay-Sachs in America, and only one child with the disease was born in Israel.

> " **Some futurists suggest that in vitro screening for obesity is no different than the use of other scientific techniques that have improved on what nature provided.** "

Ashkenazi Jewish couples are tested before marriage to determine whether they are carriers. Both parents must carry the mutated gene for the disease to be passed on; if both are carriers, there is a 25 percent chance their child will be born with Tay-Sachs. Given those odds, many Jewish couples who learn they are both carriers have elected not to have children. Says Cowan, "In the case of Tay-Sachs, a devastating genetic disease was defeated in large part by the ethnic community that was plagued by it."[29]

Testing Embryos

One test that is becoming more common is performed on embryos prior to in vitro fertilization. The preimplantation genetic diagnosis (PGD) is common among couples who have tested positive for mutated genes that cause sickle-cell anemia and breast cancer. Instead of conceiving naturally, couples conceive through in vitro fertilization. During in vitro fertilization, an egg withdrawn surgically from the mother is fertilized in a lab dish with the father's sperm. Following fertilization, the egg divides and forms an embryo, which is then implanted in the mother's uterus.

Using PGD, a fertilized embryo with as few as four cells can be tested for mutated genes. If the embryo tests negative, it is implanted in the woman. If it tests positive, parents often instruct the in vitro physician to discard the embryo.

While couples who undergo PGD do not face decisions about terminating pregnancies, critics find PGD carries the same ethical issues as eugenics. After all, they argue, parents are making decisions about creating a life based on the genetic makeup of the child. "I think it does raise some ethical questions about eugenics—selecting the genetic type of an individual,"[30] says Clint Joiner, a physician and specialist in sickle-cell anemia in Cincinnati, Ohio, who nevertheless believes PGD should remain an option for prospective parents.

Designer Babies

Within five years it is believed that PGD could be used to screen not only for disease, but for other conditions as well, such as obesity. Critics worry that if parents are led to believe their child would face a lifetime of issues stemming from obesity, they may choose not to go through with in vitro fertilization. On the other hand, some futurists suggest that in vitro screening for obesity is no different than the use of other scientific techniques that have improved on what nature provided. "Why should we think that the human genome is a once-and-for-all-finished, untamperable product?" argues Ronald M. Green, a professor of ethics at Dartmouth College in New Hampshire. "All of the biblically derived faiths permit human beings to improve on nature using technology, from agriculture to aviation. Why not improve our genome?"[31]

The moral and ethical arguments over prenatal genetic testing are complicated. Many abortion opponents are likely to consider the discarding of an egg fertilized in vitro as an act similar to the termination of a pregnancy. Yet abortion and the discarding of eggs after positive PGD tests remain part of the fabric of American life. Both procedures are among the alternatives offered to parents when faced with the sad news that a prenatal genetic test has uncovered a mutated gene.

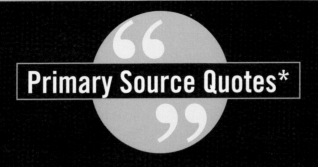

Primary Source Quotes*

How Does Genetic Testing Influence Family Planning?

66 Ten years ago, I made a decision to continue a pregnancy that would lead to a child born with Down syndrome. . . . We chose Naia, our first child, after painfully honest exchanges and much prayer.99

—Tierney Fairchild, "The Choice to be Pro-Life," *Roanoke (VA) Times*, November 10, 2008.

Fairchild's amniocentesis revealed a mutant gene that would mean her child would be born with Down syndrome; Fairchild and her husband, Greg, elected to continue the pregnancy.

66 When the fateful phone call came, I realised I had already, albeit unwittingly, taken the decision to have an abortion if my baby had Down's syndrome when I insisted on the test. I was thus prepared for it in a way perhaps others are not. And I think maybe they should be.99

—Julia Langdon and Shelley Thoupos, "Would You Abort a Baby with Down's Syndrome?" *Daily Mail (London)*,
October 28, 2009.

Langdon, who is quoted here, terminated her pregnancy after learning that her baby would be born with Down syndrome. Coauthor Thoupos elected to give birth after prenatal testing revealed her baby would be born with Down syndrome.

* Editor's Note: While the definition of a primary source can be narrowly or broadly defined, for the purposes of Compact Research, a primary source consists of: 1) results of original research presented by an organization or researcher; 2) eyewitness accounts of events, personal experience, or work experience; 3) first-person editorials offering pundits' opinions; 4) government officials presenting political plans and/or policies; 5) representatives of organizations presenting testimony or policy.

❝ If we understand the genetic cause of obesity, for example, we can intervene by means of embryo selection to produce a child with a reduced genetic likelihood of getting fat. . . . No child would have to face a lifetime of dieting or experience the health and cosmetic problems associated with obesity. **❞**

—Ronald M. Green, "Building Baby from the Genes Up," *Washington Post*, April 13, 2008. www.washingtonpost.com.

Green is a professor of ethics at Dartmouth College in New Hampshire.

❝ Consumers appear ready to use biotechnologies to test for life altering and threatening medical conditions like mental retardation, blindness, deafness, cancer, heart disease, dwarfism and shortened lifespan . . . but what they're not interested in is prenatal genetic testing to screen for traits like tall stature, superior athletic ability and superior intelligence. **❞**

—George Dvorsky, "Most Parents Not Quite Ready to Have 'Designer Babies'—but Demand Exists," Institute for Ethics and Emerging Technologies, January 28, 2009. http://ieet.org.

Dvorsky is a board member of the Institute for Ethics and Emerging Technologies, an organization based in Hartford, Connecticut, that studies the impact of science on society.

❝ Where will PGD go next? . . . Tests for a wider array of genetic characteristics, including more nonmedical ones, will be offered. One U.S. clinic already advertises on its web site that tests for hair and eye color are 'coming soon.' **❞**

—Jesse Reynolds, "Custom-Designed Kids: How Darwin's Legacy Is Being Abused," Center for Genetics and Society, February 12, 2009. www.geneticsandsociety.org.

Reynolds is the director of biotechnology accountability for the Center for Genetics and Society, a California-based organization that studies the applicability of genetic science to human life and society.

66 Genetic screening increases reproductive choice, and it also provides hope, hope that many parents never had before—hope of having, not a perfect child, but a child who, at least at the start of life, is free of devastating disease or overwhelming disability. 99

—Ruth Schwartz Cowan, *Heredity and Hope: The Case for Genetic Screening*. Cambridge, MA: Harvard University Press, 2008.

Cowan is a professor of sociology at the University of Pennsylvania in Philadelphia.

66 Women in this situation felt anxious and scared when learning of the [Down syndrome] diagnosis, and about half felt rushed or pressured into making a decision about continuing the pregnancy. . . . Combine this predisposition with the perceived 'burden' of raising a child with Down syndrome, and many women could convince themselves that abortion is their most prudent 'choice.' 99

—Susan W. Enouen, "Down Syndrome and Abortion," *Life Issues Connector*, January 2007. www.lifeissues.org.

Enouen, a resident of Cincinnati, Ohio, is an abortion opponent and columnist for *Life Issues Connector*, a publication of the Cincinnati-based Life Issues Institute, which opposes abortion rights.

66 One might conclude that where a child is deprived of sight, hearing, speech, movement, understanding, and discernment, as children with Tay-Sachs . . . are, God has declined to do His part. [Genetic] testing provides a peek at which couples will have these God-forsaken children. 99

—Masha Gessen, *Blood Matters: From Inherited Illness to Designer Babies, How the World and I Found Ourselves in the Future of the Gene*. New York: Harcourt, 2008.

Gessen, a Russian-born journalist, underwent a double mastectomy after learning she carries mutations of the genes that cause breast cancer.

"Since prenatal genetic tests don't test for every possible flaw, you have to know in advance what you're looking for. . . . An accurate and current family medical history is as important a prerequisite for prenatal testing as it is for susceptibility-gene testing.**"**

—Doris Teichler Zallen, *To Test or Not to Test*. New Brunswick, NJ: Rutgers University Press, 2008.

Zallen is a professor of science and technology in society at Virginia Tech University.

"Like sex selection, contemporary eugenics in mainstream medicine depends largely on the destruction of the 'unfit' before birth.**"**

—Maynard V. Olson, in Jan A. Witkowski and John R. Inglis, eds., *Davenport's Dream: 21st Century Reflections on Heredity and Eugenics*. Cold Spring Harbor, NY: Cold Spring Harbor Laboratory, 2008.

Olson is a professor of genome sciences at the University of Washington–Seattle.

How Does Genetic Testing Influence Family Planning?

- The Virginia law that empowered a **mental institution** to have Carrie Buck sterilized was not repealed until 1974.

- Following the U.S. Supreme Court decision authorizing involuntary sterilization, as many as **60,000 mentally infirm Americans were sterilized** against their wishes before the practice ended following World War II.

- **Seventy percent** of all pregnant women in America undergo prenatal genetic testing.

- A study of California women found that between 2006 and 2008, **23 pregnant women** learned they were carrying children who would be afflicted with cystic fibrosis; all but 3 of those women chose to terminate their pregnancies.

- In Ireland, a predominantly Catholic country where the church steadfastly opposes abortion, **50 percent** of women who learn their children will be born with Down syndrome choose to terminate their pregnancies.

- Preimplantation genetic diagnosis can find evidence that children would be born with some **170 inherited diseases**, including Huntington's disease and sickle-cell anemia.

Testing Embryos for Genetic Abnormalities

Through preimplantation genetic diagnosis (PGD) doctors can test an embryo for genetic abnormalities before it is implanted in the uterus. PGD can help ensure healthy pregnancies for women who have had multiple miscarriages and for couples who may be carriers of genetic disorders. Critics worry, however, that the procedure may also be used as a way to weed out the ill and infirm and ultimately allow people to select the traits they wish their children to have.

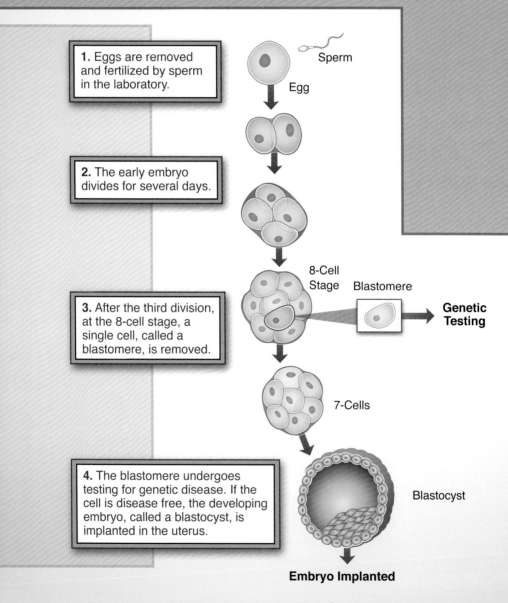

1. Eggs are removed and fertilized by sperm in the laboratory.

Sperm

Egg

2. The early embryo divides for several days.

8-Cell Stage   Blastomere

Genetic Testing

3. After the third division, at the 8-cell stage, a single cell, called a blastomere, is removed.

7-Cells

4. The blastomere undergoes testing for genetic disease. If the cell is disease free, the developing embryo, called a blastocyst, is implanted in the uterus.

Blastocyst

Embryo Implanted

Source: Laurie Tarkan, "Screening for Abnormal Embryos Offer Couples Hope After Heartbreak," *New York Times*, November 22, 2005. www.nytimes.com.

Some Genetic Disorders That Can Be Detected Before Birth

Prenatal diagnostic testing can determine whether a fetus has certain abnormalities. Some of these tests are considered part of routine prenatal care. Others are done when couples have an increased risk of having a baby with a genetic abnormality. Factors that affect increased risk include the age of the parents, family history of a disease, and racial or ethnic background of the parents.

Disorder	Incidence
Cystic fibrosis	1 of 3,300 white people
Congenital adrenal hyperplasia	1 of 10,000
Duchenne muscular dystrophy	1 of 3,500 male births
Hemophilia A	1 of 8,500 male births
Alpha- and beta-thalassemia	Varies widely by ethnic and racial group
Fragile X syndrome	1 of 2,000 male births 1 of 4,000 female births
Polycystic kidney disease (adult type)	1 of 3,000
Sickle-cell anemia	1 of 400 black people in the United States
Tay-Sachs disease	1 of 3,600 Ashkenazi Jews and French Canadians 1 of 400,000 in other groups

Source: *Merck Manual Home Edition*, "Genetic Disorders Detection: Prenatal Diagnostic Testing," 2008. www.merck.com.

- About 5,500 American children are born with Down syndrome each year; according to the National Down Syndrome Society, there are some **400,000 people living with Down syndrome** in the United States.

- A study published in the journal *Prenatal Testing and Disability Rights* found that **23 percent** of physicians encourage women whose prenatal tests reveal Down syndrome to undergo abortions.

- A poll conducted by Johns Hopkins University in Baltimore, Maryland, found that **two-thirds** of Americans support the use of preimplantation genetic diagnosis to prevent childhood diseases.

- According to Reprogenetics, a New Jersey company that provides in vitro fertilizations, as many as **5 percent** of preimplantation genetic diagnoses fail to identify defects in embryos that could lead to inherited diseases.

- Prior to the commencement of Tay-Sachs testing, about **50 to 60 babies** were born each year with the disease; in 2003 no American baby was born with Tay-Sachs and only 1 Israeli child was born with the disease.

Will Genetic Testing Lead to Discrimination?

> **66**We are living through an era of the ascendance of biology, and we have to be very careful. We will all be walking a fine line between using biology and allowing it to be abused.**99**
>
> —Henry Louis Gates Jr., author, scholar, and director of the W.E.B. Du Bois Institute for African and African American Research at Harvard University.

> **66**The message to employees is they should now be able to get whatever genetic counseling or testing they need and be less fearful about doing so.**99**
>
> —Peggy R. Mastroianni, associate legal counsel for the U.S. Equal Employment Opportunity Commission.

Suspicions About Screening

While it would seem as though genetic testing would be universally embraced as an important step forward in detecting diseases, that has not been the case. As medical researchers made their earliest breakthroughs, many individuals and groups harbored doubts and suspicions about the science, believing that genetic information could be used for much darker purposes.

By 1972 a genetic test had been developed to detect sickle-cell anemia, a disease largely confined to people of African descent. As screening programs were launched in African American communities, leaders of the Black Panther Party voiced strenuous objections. The Black Panthers were regarded as a radical group, but the organization held tremendous influence over many inner-city black citizens.

Panther leaders were suspicious of the tests, suggesting that white political leaders had set up phony screening programs that would fail to detect the disease, thereby guaranteeing carriers would continue to produce offspring afflicted with sickle-cell anemia. Said one Panther publication: "Sickle cell anemia is a deadly blood disease that is peculiar to black people. . . . The racist U.S. power structure has no intention of ceasing this form of genocide since it is this racist power structure that perpetuates the disease."[32]

> As medical researchers made their earliest breakthroughs, many individuals and groups harbored doubts and suspicions about the science, believing that genetic information could be used for much darker purposes.

Instead the Panthers advocated a blood test for sickle-cell anemia that did not rely on genetics, even setting up their own clinics to administer the screenings. The test the Panthers urged people to undergo was regarded as far less accurate than genetic screening. Therefore it is likely that by campaigning against DNA testing, the Panthers may have been partly responsible for helping to perpetuate a disease they hoped to wipe out.

The Search for the "Gay Gene"

For decades sociologists have speculated on the roots of homosexuality: Do homosexuals decide, at some point in their lives, to embrace a gay lifestyle? Or are people born gay? Is homosexuality hardwired into their DNA?

In 1993 genetics researcher Dean Hamer believed he had found the answer, publishing a paper that identified a specific gene—found only on the male chromosome—that he suggested serves as a trigger for homosexuality. Hamer's findings were disputed by other scientists who claimed he limited his research to acknowledged homosexual men. They suggested a much wider study might show the gene might be found on the chromosomes of heterosexuals as well. "A frequent criticism of Hamer's paper was that he did not measure the incidence of [genetic] markers among heterosexual brothers of gay sibling pairs," said Richard Horton, editor of the British medical journal the *Lancet*. "Without this information, it is impossible to guess the influence of any genes."[33]

Over the years, the scientific debate over the existence of the gay gene has never been settled. In the meantime, leaders of the gay community have raised alarms that if, indeed, a gay gene is identified, it is possible that genetic information could be used as a basis for discrimination against homosexuals. Says John DeCecco, a psychology professor at San Francisco State University and editor of the *Journal of Homosexuality*, "One imagines a pregnant mother and father being told, 'Your baby is going to be queer. Do you want it?'"[34]

Fears of Discrimination

With the completion of the projects to map the human genome in 2003, genetic testing became more specific—new tests were developed to identify mutant genes that could cause hundreds of diseases. Doctors expected the demand for gene testing to increase, but patients did not flock to their offices. Many who did undergo the tests asked that the results be kept private.

Doctors found that people did not want their insurance companies or employers to know the results of their genetic tests. They feared discrimination in the workplace or a loss of insurance benefits. "It's pretty clear that the public is afraid of taking advantage of genetic testing," said Francis S. Collins, director of the National Human Genome Research Institute, which headed the public project to map the human genome. "If that continues, the future of medicine that we would all like to see happen stands the chance of being dead on arrival."[35]

The completion of the projects to map the human genome came amid an era when health insurance companies were likely to reject applicants for insurance if they were afflicted with preexisting conditions. It was very difficult, for example, for an uninsured cancer patient to buy insurance because the insurance company would know it would likely have to cover expensive treatment costs for the patient.

Could a genetic predisposition for disease be considered a preexisting condition? Victoria Grove, of Woodbury, Minnesota, was one person who found herself caught between the need to know the composition of her DNA and the need to keep that information secret. Several of Grove's family members were afflicted with emphysema, a crippling lung disease. Grove feared that if she went to a doctor for a genetic test, she would be unable to afford health insurance because existence of the mutant gene would show up in her records. "Something needs to be done so that you cannot be discriminated against when you know about these things,"[36] she said.

No Discrimination on the Basis of Genetics

Prompted by fears of discrimination, Congress passed the Genetic Information Nondiscrimination Act (GINA) in 2008, prohibiting discrimination by health insurance companies and employers due to the existence of long-dormant genes that could render the patient ill. The law prohibits health insurance companies from using genetic information to deny coverage or raise fees for individuals who buy their own insurance or for employers who offer health insurance as a workplace benefit. The law also bars employers from collecting genetic information from employees or job applicants and using that information in making decisions on hiring, firing, and salaries.

"This is a tremendous victory for every American not born with perfect genes, which means it's a victory for every single one of us," said Louise M. Slaughter, a member of the U.S. House of Representatives from New York. "Since all of us are predisposed to at least a few genetic-based disorders, we are all potential victims of genetic discrimination."[37]

Privacy Rights vs. Predictive Genomics

Scientists predict that in the future, all people will have their genomes mapped, which will enable doctors to tell whether they have a predisposition to many diseases. But getting one's genome mapped will mean that the information has to be stored somewhere, and at this point no one seems to know where.

It also means people who get their genomes mapped may find their privacy violated if the information about their DNA is not kept secure. Experts worry about computer-savvy thieves hacking into records to obtain genetic information about individuals. Virginia Tech University professor Doris Teichler Zallen says she has encountered clients of DNA testing labs who question the security of their information. "One agitated consumer felt that any promise of genetic privacy was 'quaint,'" Zallen recalled, "that there would be no way in this computer age, with electronic records out in cyberspace, for such protections to be realistic."[38]

Thieves who gain access to human genomes could find any number of uses for the records. For example, records could be sold to drug companies or other medical providers interested in establishing databases of potential customers suffering from particular afflictions.

> " Doctors found that people did not want their insurance companies or employers to know the results of their genetic tests. They feared discrimination in the workplace or a loss of insurance benefits. "

A government-operated database containing everyone's DNA data may offer more security, but many people find the notion of the government keeping genetic records on private citizens unacceptable. "It's only a matter of time before the government gets its hands on those DNA samples and starts playing around with our genetic codes," says Barry Steinhardt, a privacy specialist for the American Civil Liberties Union. "We're not just on a slippery slope, we're halfway down it."[39]

Emergence of DNA Banks

DNA databases of criminals have existed since 1998, when Congress authorized the FBI to establish the Combined DNA Index System (CODIS). At first the use of DNA evidence was collected mostly from sex offenders and in homicide cases, but in recent years the database has been fed DNA records on all convicted criminals. By 2010 the FBI's DNA database contained profiles of nearly 8 million criminals. Federal law enforcement agencies as well as state and local police provide profiles for the database.

The FBI has made plans to expand the database to include not only convicted criminals but people who have been arrested and not yet tried as well as illegal immigrants. Indeed, in 2009 FBI officials predicted the national database of DNA evidence would grow by 80,000 profiles a month.

Law enforcement experts contend the expansion of the DNA database would greatly assist police in matching suspects to crime scenes. "DNA is to the 21st century what fingerprinting was to the 20th," said federal prosecutor Deborah Daniels. "The widespread use of DNA evidence is the future of law enforcement in this country."[40]

Critics fear the database will continue to expand and, eventually, genetic records from minor offenders will end up in CODIS. "What we object to, and what the Constitution prohibits, is the indiscriminate taking of DNA for things like writing an insufficient funds check, shoplifting and [minor] drug convictions,"[41] says American Civil Liberties Union lawyer Michael Risher.

DNA and Racial Profiling

Racial profiling has emerged as an issue in the collection of DNA. Racial profiling is used by some members of law enforcement to identify potential suspects based on race, ethnicity, nationality, or religion, rather than on evidence or suspicion of criminal behavior. Scientists do not yet agree on whether DNA can help police pinpoint race. In one celebrated case in Baton Rouge, Louisiana, however, a molecular biologist who examined a serial killer's DNA was able to direct police toward an African American suspect when, at the time, police believed the perpetrator was white. Police followed the biologist's advice, redirected their investigation, and soon made an arrest of a black suspect, who was eventually convicted.

> " Getting one's genome mapped will mean that the information has to be stored somewhere, and at this point no one seems to know where. "

DNAPrint Genomics, the Florida company that developed the racial test in the Louisiana case, says it has been able to identify genetic markers commonly found in certain population groups, including European, sub-Saharan African, Southeast Asian, and Native American.

Critics counter, though, that profiling suspects by race sets a dangerous precedent. "How far are we from having [ancestry tests] used to justify taking DNA from any black man on a street corner, because we think a Sub-Saharan African committed the crime?"[42] argues Ingrid Gill, a Chicago, Illinois, lawyer and expert on DNA evidence.

Storing DNA from Babies

The day when a comprehensive national DNA database becomes a reality may not be that far in the future. Starting in the 1990s many state governments required hospitals to draw blood from newborns to test the children for inherited diseases. Some states have opted to store these DNA records indefinitely, leading privacy advocates to question whether a database of DNA is being created.

As parents learn that their children's DNA is in storage, many have objected and filed lawsuits. In Minnesota, for example, 815,000 DNA samples are included in the state's database. One of the DNA profiles in the Minnesota database belongs to Isabel Brown.

Isabel's mother, Annie Brown, says she was told by a doctor that her infant daughter may carry a mutant gene that causes cystic fibrosis. Brown says she was shocked by the news—and also shocked that the doctor knew about Isabel's DNA because Brown and her husband did not know the girl's DNA had been tested. Further tests have indicated that Isabel does not carry the mutant gene. Still, Brown says the state should not have taken her daughter's DNA without the family's permission. Says Brown: "Why do they need to store my baby's DNA indefinitely? Something on there could affect her ability to get a job later on, or get health insurance."[43]

> " As parents learn that their children's DNA is in storage, many have objected and filed lawsuits.

While it would seem as though the federal government has taken steps to ensure that nobody would be denied health insurance or employment based on the content of their DNA, there are still many issues about privacy and discrimination that remain unresolved. And as genetic testing becomes more widespread and more records are collected on more people, these issues are sure to remain as troubling shadows over the world of genetic science.

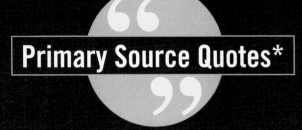

Primary Source Quotes*

Will Genetic Testing Lead to Discrimination?

66 People should not lose their medical insurance when genetic tests show they are at risk for illnesses. It is not their fault if they will have greater medical costs. Logically, they should be insured against genetic problems before they are born. That's what insurance is for—to avoid having to bear large costs because of circumstances beyond one's control. 99

—Fred E. Foldvary, "Must We Subsidize Genetic Flaws?" *Progress Report*, May 2008. www.progress.org.

Foldvary is a lecturer in economics at Santa Clara University in California.

66 Because of what was once said about sickle cell screening, African Americans remain one of the demographic groups least likely to participate in any form of genetic testing. . . . Bitter memories, in this case, trumped concerns about individual and community health. 99

—Ruth Schwartz Cowan, *Heredity and Hope: The Case for Genetic Screening*. Cambridge, MA: Harvard University Press, 2008.

Cowan is a professor of sociology at the University of Pennsylvania in Philadelphia.

Bracketed quotes indicate conflicting positions.

* Editor's Note: While the definition of a primary source can be narrowly or broadly defined, for the purposes of Compact Research, a primary source consists of: 1) results of original research presented by an organization or researcher; 2) eyewitness accounts of events, personal experience, or work experience; 3) first-person editorials offering pundits' opinions; 4) government officials presenting political plans and/or policies; 5) representatives of organizations presenting testimony or policy.

66 I suspect many laypersons will wildly cheer such legislation, as yet another way to 'get tough' on criminals and prevent crime.... It is, however, more than a little troubling that [lawmakers] would cavalierly dismiss the serious constitutional concerns embedded in a law mandating that a person not convicted of any offense whatsoever should be forced to surrender their DNA to the government. 99

—Bob Barr, "DNA Database Bill Should Be Deep-Sixed," *Atlanta Journal-Constitution*, February 8, 2010. http://blogs.ajc.com.

Barr is a former member of Congress from Georgia and the Libertarian Party candidate for president in 2008.

66 We need a more robust DNA database, available to law enforcement in every state, to continue to tighten the grip around folks who have perpetrated these crimes. But critics have a point that genetic police work, like the sampling of arrestees, is fraught with bias. A better solution: to keep every American's DNA profile on file. 99

—Michael Seringhaus, "To Stop Crime, Share Your Genes," *New York Times*, March 15, 2010.

Seringhaus is editor of the *Yale Journal of Law and Technology* and the holder of a doctorate in molecular biophysics.

66 Banning genetic discrimination in insurance may also have bad consequences, owing to the phenomenon of adverse selection. Suppose that you undergo a genetic test showing that you have very 'safe' genes—you are not predisposed to any serious diseases. If your health insurer cannot genetically discriminate, you will be charged the same premium as higher risk individuals. 99

—Tom Douglas, "Genetic Discrimination and the Future of Health Insurance," *Practical Ethics*, May 1, 2008. www.practicalethicsnews.com.

A doctoral student at the University of Oxford in England, Douglas is studying medical ethics and psychology.

66 GINA, the first civil rights legislation of this century, will stamp out a form of discrimination while also allowing us to realize the tremendous life-saving and life-altering potential of genetic research. The important protections assured by GINA will enable the scientific and medical communities to make the critical medical breakthroughs of the 21st century. **99**

—U.S. representative Louise M. Slaughter, "Genetic Information Nondiscrimination Act," February 26, 2008.
www.louise.house.gov.

A member of the U.S. House of Representatives, Slaughter represents a congressional district in northern New York State.

66 [GINA] applies only to two aspects of the problem, discrimination in health insurance and employment. . . . GINA does nothing to prohibit discrimination in life insurance, disability insurance, long-term care insurance, mortgages, commercial transactions, or any of the other possible uses of genetic information. **99**

—Mark A. Rothstein, "GINA's Beauty Is Only Skin Deep," *Gene Watch*, April/May 2009.
www.councilforresponsiblegenetics.org.

Rothstein is the director of the Institute for Bioethics, Health Policy and Law at the University of Louisville School of Medicine in Kentucky.

66 Given the racial disparities in our criminal justice system—particularly with regard to racial profiling and who is arrested in the first place—you can wind up with a DNA database that not only fails to serve the public safety, but that is also a discriminatory boondoggle because it over represents minorities and the poor. **99**

—Courtenay Strickland, "Dexter, DNA and Your Privacy," American Civil Liberties Union, November 25, 2009.
www.aclu.org.

Strickland is the director of public policy and advocacy for the American Civil Liberties Union of Florida.

66 If people at risk for inherited diseases are unwilling to undergo genetic testing, they forego information of potentially immense importance to their lives. And if that same mistrust prevents citizens from participating in genetic and genomic research, the process by which our society develops new medicines and cures will suffer. 99

—Misha Angrist and Robert Cook-Deegan, "Nice to Meet You, GINA: I've Heard So Much About You," Duke University Institute for Genome Sciences and Policy, May 9, 2008. www.genome.duke.edu.

Angrist is an assistant professor at the Duke University Institute for Genome Sciences and Policy in North Carolina; Cook-Deegan is the director of the institute's Center for Genome Ethics, Law and Policy.

Will Genetic Testing Lead to Discrimination?

- The **Genetic Information Nondiscrimination Act** was passed by a unanimous vote in the Senate and with just a single dissenting vote in the House of Representatives.

- A poll commissioned by Johns Hopkins University in Baltimore, Maryland, found that **92 percent** of respondents believe their genetic information can somehow be used against them.

- Prior to the adoption of the Genetic Information Nondiscrimination Act, New York–Presbyterian/Weill Cornell Medical Center reported that **20 percent** of patients taking a genetic test for breast cancer chose to pay for the test with **cash to avoid submitting the bills to their insurance companies** out of fear that the insurers would learn the results.

- A U.S. Department of Labor study found that **63 percent** of workers said they would refuse to take genetic tests if they knew their employers would see the results.

- To settle a lawsuit filed by its employees, the Burlington Northern Railroad was forced to pay **$2.2 million** to 36 workers who were compelled to submit to DNA tests; the employees alleged in the suit that the railroad wanted to know if they were genetically predisposed to disabilities.

The National DNA Database

Genetic testing has given law enforcement an invaluable tool for solving crimes, but civil libertarians worry that DNA profiles of many innocent people, such as those arrested but not convicted of crimes, may be misused. DNA profiles of nearly 8 million people are kept in a national database maintained by the FBI. The database includes records of convicted felons from nearly all states. Some states also send the FBI the DNA profiles of juveniles, arrestees, illegal immigrants, and people convicted of misdemeanors. How that information is used by law enforcement is of growing concern.

All Felons

47 states and federal agencies

Some Misdemeanor Offenders

16 states

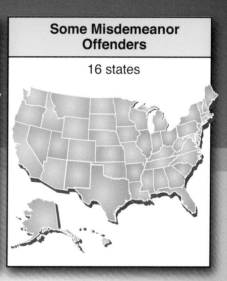

Some Arrestees

15 states and federal agencies

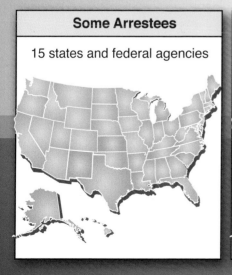

Some Juveniles

35 states

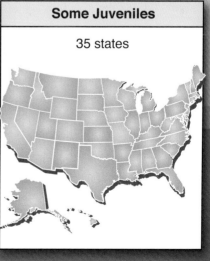

Discrimination Fears and the "Gay Gene"

Americans have long debated whether homosexuality is an inborn trait or the result of upbringing and environment. According to a 2008 poll, 42 percent of Americans believe that homosexuality is something people are born with—a marked contrast with opinions expressed in earlier polls. Science has never actually proven the existence of a "gay gene," but if it were shown to exist, leaders in the gay community worry that it could be used as a basis for discrimination against homosexuals.

Question: In your view, is homosexuality something a person is born with or is homosexuality due to other factors such as upbringing and environment?

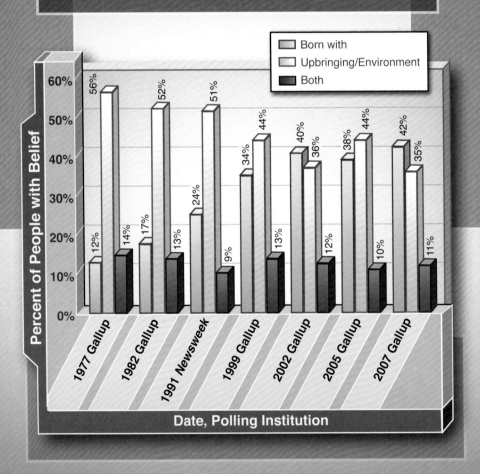

Source: Karlyn Bowmans, "Attitudes About Homosexuality and Gay Marriage," American Enterprise Institute, June 3, 2008. www.aei.org.

- Most states mandate that newborn babies be tested for up to **58 separate diseases and disorders**, including many inherited conditions.

- More than **20 scientific studies** of genetics have been produced since 2000 using the data collected from genetic tests performed on newborns.

- A database maintained by British police contains the DNA profiles of **77 percent** of the country's male black population between the ages of 15 and 34; in contrast, the database includes DNA profiles of just **22 percent** of the white male population in the same age group.

- The British police database includes DNA profiles of **750,000** children as well as the profiles of **340,000** people who were arrested but cleared of wrongdoing, and **20,000** profiles of people who provided DNA samples during investigations but were ultimately not arrested.

- During the next few years, the FBI's national database of DNA is expected to grow by **80,000 profiles per month**.

What Is the Future of Genetic Testing?

> **❝I was devastated. You find out you've been taking this medication for all this time, and find out you are not getting any benefit.❞**
>
> —Jody Uslan, a California woman whose test revealed that due to her genetic makeup, the drug she took to prevent the recurrence of breast cancer had no effect.

> **❝The goal of personalized medicine is to get the best medical outcomes by choosing treatments that work well with a person's genomic profile.❞**
>
> —Felix Frueh, associate director of genomics for the U.S. Food and Drug Administration.

The Emergence of Personalized Medicine

When Cecily Harris was diagnosed with lung cancer, doctors told the woman from Englewood, New Jersey, to expect the worst. Harris's cancer was particularly aggressive, producing a large tumor in her lung. Doctors gave her nine months to live. Harris defied the odds with the help of the drug Iressa. Unlike other anticancer drugs, Iressa does not kill cancerous cells but instead binds itself to a chemical in the cells that enhances their growth. When Iressa is administered, the drug sends a signal to the chemical, turning it off.

Iressa may sound like a miracle drug, but that is not the case. The drug works in about 10 percent of lung cancer patients only—those who are carriers of a mutated gene that enables the drug to perform its work, turning off the growth switch in the cancerous cells. Harris was prescribed Iressa after a genetic test revealed the presence of the gene mutation. Now, more than a decade after receiving her dim prognosis, Harris has beaten her cancer. "I feel as well as a 76-year-old can feel," she says. "I'm one of the lucky ones."[44]

In Harris's case, doctors employed a therapy known as pharmacogenomics: They administered a drug according to the genetic makeup of the patient. As patients undergo genetic testing, doctors will be able to prescribe drugs that work in concert with their genes. Medicine will become "personalized." Says Charles J. Lusch, a cancer specialist in Reading, Pennsylvania, "Now is the age of targeted therapy, and it's exploding."[45]

> **The drug works in about 10 percent of lung cancer patients only—those who are carriers of a mutated gene that enables the drug to perform its work, turning off the growth switch in the cancerous cells.**

Harris's case illustrates how genetic testing is on the brink of expanding to a much wider segment of the community. For years the testing has been confined mostly to people who have reason to suspect they might get sick because an illness is common in their families or to expectant mothers who believe their babies may be born with diseases or disabilities. Soon a much wider variety of patients may benefit from therapies based on genetic testing.

Customized Drugs

The addition of the drug warfarin to the list of pharmacogenomic drugs is regarded as a major breakthrough in the treatment of patients who are at risk for heart attacks and strokes. Warfarin is a blood-thinning agent that prevents clots that could clog arteries. About 4 million Americans take the drug. For years, though, the administration of warfarin has been hit-and-miss as doctors were forced to guess at the proper doses.

Giving a patient the wrong dosage of warfarin could be dangerous: too little and the drug does no good; too much and the drug could cause internal bleeding and even be fatal. In recent years researchers have found they could tailor the dose of warfarin based on the patient's genetic makeup. "You can give the standard dose of warfarin and some people are just fine, while others have significant complications such as bleeding in the brain," says genetic researcher Michael Caldwell. "If you identify a patient's genetic makeup, we can get a better handle on the appropriate dose."[46]

Researchers have found two common genes that affect a patient's response to warfarin. One gene governs how well the drug is absorbed into the patient's blood, and the other governs the patient's sensitivity to the drug. By looking at the variations in the two genes, doctors believe they can provide patients with the proper amount of warfarin.

Pharmacogenomics has another application: In addition to telling people which drug is right for them, the science can also tell people which drugs are wrong. For example, in recent years some breast cancer patients have learned through genetic testing that the drug tamoxifen has not been helping to prevent the recurrences of their cancers. Researchers have discovered that the drug is effective only in people whose genes produce a chemical that enables the drug to work. Therefore, the researchers concluded, as many as 7 percent of tamoxifen patients have been getting no benefit from the drug because they lack the key gene. "There's a subset of people that benefit and a subset of people that doesn't," said Herbert K. Lyerly, a breast cancer specialist at Duke University in North Carolina. "This has profound implications for how we develop drugs and how we use them."[47]

Direct-to-Consumer Genetic Testing

By 2010 it was becoming clear that a patient need not go to a doctor to obtain a genetic test. Many companies had entered the direct-to-consumer field. For fees that are often less than $100, people can mail saliva or blood samples to private companies and in a few weeks receive reports containing many details about themselves, including their predisposition to develop diseases.

Experts are wary of direct-to-consumer tests, arguing that medical professionals should help people interpret the results. (Some direct-to-consumer companies provide assistance on a limited basis, usually over the phone.) Many experts fear people may misinterpret the results of their tests. "My personal opinion is these tests are a waste of money," says genetic counselor Christine Patch. "[The test] doesn't tell them very much and it may tell them the wrong thing."[48]

In 2010 a California company, Pathway Genomics, announced plans to stock nonprescription direct-to-consumer genetic tests on the shelves of the CVS and Walgreens drugstore chains. The kit would cost $20 in the store, but other fees would be charged when the consumer mailed the sample to the company. Depending on what the consumer asks to be tested for, the fees could range from $79 to $399.

The U.S. Food and Drug Administration asked Pathway to delay sales of the test, and the company agreed. The Food and Drug Administration announced it plans to examine the entire direct-to-consumer genetic test industry to determine whether the tests should be regarded as medical devices and therefore subject to strict regulations.

Testing for Gender

Direct-to-consumer testing can be used to find out more than just a patient's predisposition to developing a disease. The tests can also be employed to determine the gender of a fetus. That is what Carey Peacock had in mind when she obtained a direct-to-consumer DNA test after learning she was pregnant. Peacock had already given birth to a boy and desperately wanted a daughter. She could have learned the gender through a routine ultrasound test, but that test is typically administered in the sixteenth week of pregnancy and Peacock wanted to know sooner. A week after mailing in a sample of her DNA, Peacock got the news: She would be giving birth to another boy. "I love my two boys so fiercely," Peacock said after the birth of her second child, "[but] some days I think my family isn't complete yet."[49]

Given the desire by many parents to know the genders of the fetuses as soon as possible, some direct-to-

> " For fees that are often less than $100, people can mail saliva or blood samples to private companies and in a few weeks receive reports containing many details about themselves, including their predisposition to develop diseases. "

> **Some laboratories that perform pre-implantation diagnosis tests will, if the parents request it, separate out the male or female chromosomes from the father's DNA before performing the in vitro fertilization.**

consumer companies are specializing in predicting gender. One California company, Consumer Genetics, has named its test Tell Me Pink or Blue.

Like Peacock, many parents accept the news even if the tests tell them they will not get the gender they had hoped for, but some experts fear that early testing for gender raises the notion that parents might opt for abortions rather than deliver children whose gender they refuse to accept. Says Kathy Hudson, director of the Washington, D.C.–based Genetics and Public Policy Center, which examines the impact of genetic science on society: "The question is, 'How are people going to use that information?' I think it would be troubling if people were selectively terminating pregnancies based on gender."[50]

Genetic Testing and Gender Selection

Not only is it possible for parents to learn the genders of their babies long before the births, but actually selecting the gender of the child is now possible through in vitro fertilization. Some laboratories that perform pre-implantation diagnosis tests will, if the parents request it, separate out the male or female chromosomes from the father's DNA before performing the in vitro fertilization. This process is believed to provide a high probability that a child would be born in the gender selected by the parents.

Jeffrey Steinberg, director of the Fertility Institutes, a California in vitro clinic that offers sex selection, says there is a large demand among parents who want to select the gender of their children. "We've seen a huge international onslaught of people that are just interested in balancing their families,"[51] says Steinberg.

Other doctors counter that gender selection goes beyond the scope of what preimplantation diagnosis was intended to do: detect evidence of disease in the DNA of an embryo. Mark Hughes, a physician who helped pioneer preimplantation diagnosis, says he sees parents opting for in vitro fertilization even though it is clear they are not having trouble conceiving naturally and instead are simply interested in picking the gender of their children. "I went into medicine to diagnose and treat and hopefully cure disease," says Hughes. "Your gender is not a disease, last time I checked. . . . There's no suffering. There's no illness. And I don't think doctors have any business being there."[52]

Finding New Redheads

Direct-to-consumer genetic tests can provide people with more than just health-related information. Many private companies are already offering home DNA tests that can help people learn about their ancestries. By examining people's DNA, companies can help clients trace their roots—telling them, for example, the region of Europe, Africa, or Asia where their ancestors lived.

This information is helping some people solve mysteries about themselves. Dark-complexioned, Wayne Joseph grew up in Louisiana believing he was African American—although he suspected some measure of mixed ancestry in his blood. After taking a home DNA test, Joseph was shocked at the results. The test showed he was 57 percent European, 39 percent Native American, and 4 percent Asian. None of his ancestors, it turned out, were from Africa. "I was floored,"[53] he says.

As home DNA genetic testing gains in popularity, the companies that offer the tests are finding they can provide more information that people may find of interest. For example, one California company, Alpha Biolaboratory, specializes in testing people to determine whether they will produce babies

> " Francis Crick, one of the molecular biologists who discovered the structure of DNA, underwent genetic testing but said he had no interest in knowing the results. When Crick died in 2004, the cause of death was colon cancer—a condition that can be predicted through genetic testing. "

with red hair—a source of pride among redheads who worry that the trait of red hair is being diluted through intermarriage.

The "redhead" gene, known as MC1R, is recessive, meaning both parents must pass on the gene to the child in order for the baby to be born with red hair. "We started getting requests from people who wanted to know if they inherited the red hair trait, what might be the chance of having a redheaded baby," says Tzung-Fu Hsieh, a genetic scientist who helped develop the "red tracer" DNA test for Alpha Biolaboratory. "So we've known for awhile that some people were looking for such a service."[54]

The Right Not to Know

Although genetic testing can provide people with answers about their futures, many people prefer not to know. They are comfortable with life as they know it and see no reason to live in a state of dread or panic if told that, at some point in the future, they are likely to develop an unfortunate disease. Indeed, Francis Crick, one of the the molecular biologists who discovered the structure of DNA, underwent genetic testing but said he had no interest in knowing the results. When Crick died in 2004, the cause of death was colon cancer—a condition that can be predicted through genetic testing.

As genetic testing becomes more widespread, there are many issues yet to be resolved, such as whether direct-to-consumer testing is accurate and whether personalized medicine, gene therapy, and gender selection become the new standards of medicine. First, though, it is clear that many people will find themselves making very difficult decisions about whether they truly want to know what the future may hold for them.

What Is the Future of Genetic Testing?

66 **Those who arrange all the testing on their own can find themselves at the mercy of direct-to-consumer organizations, some of which may be out for a quick profit and not organized to deliver high-quality services or to provide effective follow-up recommendations.** 99

—Doris Teichler Zallen, *To Test or Not to Test*. New Brunswick, NJ: Rutgers University Press, 2008.

Zallen is a professor of science and technology in society at Virginia Tech University.

66 **So was it worth the money? It was alarming to learn that I have a far greater risk of macular degeneration, an age-related eye disorder that results in loss of central vision . . . and 13 times the average risk for getting glaucoma. I shall now be watchful for early signs. I shall also discuss with my general practitioner anything I could be doing—or taking—to reduce the risk.** 99

—Cassandra Jardine, "A Dip in the Gene Pool Reveals What I'm Made Of," *Daily Telegraph*, June 2, 2008.

Jardine is a columnist for the *Daily Telegraph*, a newspaper based in London, England.

* Editor's Note: While the definition of a primary source can be narrowly or broadly defined, for the purposes of Compact Research, a primary source consists of: 1) results of original research presented by an organization or researcher; 2) eyewitness accounts of events, personal experience, or work experience; 3) first-person editorials offering pundits' opinions; 4) government officials presenting political plans and/or policies; 5) representatives of organizations presenting testimony or policy.

❝Parents may wish to have a child of a specific sex, generally male, and be willing to terminate the pregnancy to have the preferred child. To put it bluntly, they do want a child, but do not want that particular one. Sex selection is gender discrimination.❞

—Evelyne Shuster, "Sex Selection Is Gender Discrimination," Opposing Views, December 10, 2008. www.opposingviews.com.

Shuster is a medical ethicist for the Veterans Affairs Medical Center in Philadelphia, Pennsylvania.

❝Would permitting sex selection further increase males' advantages over females in society? To address this concern and minimize the problem, programs that offer sex selection can require parents requesting the service to have had at least one child of the opposite sex. This places the emphasis on family balancing, rather than meeting parents' sex preference.❞

—Ronald M. Green, *Babies by Design: The Ethics of Genetic Choice*. New Haven, CT: Yale University Press, 2008.

Green is a professor of ethics at Dartmouth College in New Hampshire.

❝The dawn of personal genomics promises benefits and pitfalls that no one can foresee. It could usher in an era of personalized medicine, in which drug regimens are customized for a patient's biochemistry rather than juggled through trial and error, and screening and prevention measures are aimed at those who are most at risk.❞

—Steven Pinker, "My Genome, Myself," *New York Times*, January 11, 2009.

Pinker is a professor of psychology at Harvard University.

❝Drug metabolism isn't only based on our genetic makeup, but is affected by many additional factors, such as body size and age. And, since pharmacogenomics is a relatively new science, insurance companies may not reimburse for the cost of genetic testing.❞

—Carrie A. Zabel, "Pharmacogenomics: Personalized Medicine at the Corner Drugstore," Mayo Clinic, February 24, 2010. www.mayoclinic.com.

Zabel is the genetic counselor at the Mayo Clinic, the medical center in Rochester, Minnesota, regarded as one of the top research-oriented hospitals in America.

❝The term 'personalized medicine' reflects the growth of scientific understanding and medical tools that can help individualize care at a new level. Such tools can help match treatments to individual genetic variations . . . and that can help take the guesswork out of medicine, making healthcare decisions more precise.❞

—Michael O. Levitt and Raju Kucherlapati, "The Great Promise of Personalized Medicine," *Boston Globe*, December 26, 2008. www.boston.com.

Levitt is a former secretary of the U.S. Department of Health and Human Services; Kucherlapati is a professor of genetics at Harvard University Medical School.

❝We have so many ancestors that the genetic echoes of any one ancestor get washed out over time, so someone taking [a DNA] test hoping to find proof of that Cherokee princess so many families claim is apt to be disappointed.❞

—Megan Smolenyak, "Playing with DNA: Is Larry David Really 37 Percent Native American?" *Huffington Post*, December 24, 2009. www.huffingtonpost.com.

Smolenyak is an author and expert in genealogical research who helps people trace their family trees.

Facts and Illustrations

What Is the Future of Genetic Testing?

- Prescriptions for more than **200 drugs** on the market can be tailored to the needs of individual patients based on the results of genetic tests of the patients, the U.S. Food and Drug Administration says.

- Most laboratories that perform preimplantation diagnosis tests have a **60 percent** success rate in providing parents the gender they request through in vitro fertilization, although one Virginia lab says it has a **76 percent** success rate for boys and a **91 percent** success rate for girls.

- Great Britain has **outlawed gender selection** through preimplantation diagnosis testing.

- By 2008 it was estimated that at least **30 private companies** had entered the business of direct-to-consumer genetic testing.

- By 2010 most health-related direct-to-consumer genetic tests were sold over the Internet; total sales of those kits were believed to number fewer than **100,000**.

- According to *Science* magazine, nearly **500,000** people have undergone genetic tests to help trace the geographic origins of their ancestors.

- According to the U.S. Department of Health and Human Services, providing patients with more accurate doses of warfarin through genetic testing could save patients money, for a cumulative potential savings of some **$1 billion**.

Direct-to-Consumer Genetic Tests

People are learning they do not have to go to the doctor to find out if there is something wrong with them. Many private companies offer direct-to-consumer genetic tests that will predict or even diagnose such conditions as asthma, heart disease, and cancer. Medical experts find this to be an alarming trend: They say that direct-to-consumer tests are often not accurate, nor do the companies offer adequate counseling to help patients interpret the results. One 2009 study found that 10 separate companies offered screenings for cancer while 16 offered genetic testing for heart disease.

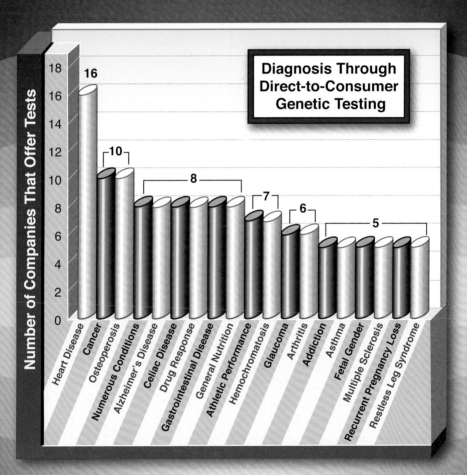

Source: T. Caulfield et al., "Direct-to-Consumer Genetic Testing: Good, Bad or Benign?" *Clinical Genetics*, 2009, p. 1.

Celebrity Genetic Tests for Ancestry

People who have questions about their ancestry are turning to genetic testing for answers. Guests on the TV talk show *Lopez Tonight* were asked to undergo DNA tests to trace their ancestries, which were revealed on the show. Some of the stars have been startled to learn the results. TV writer and comic Larry David, an Ashkenazi Jew, learned that he has 37 percent Native American blood. Others who were tested included hip-hop star Snoop Dogg, actress Jessica Alba, and former pro basketball player Charles Barkley.

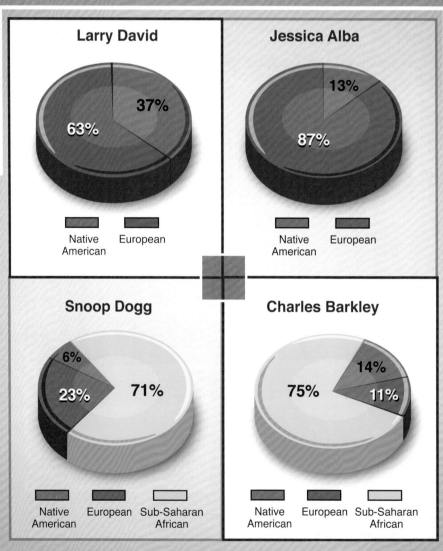

Sources: Newsletter of the International Society of Genetic Genealogy, December 2009. www.isogg.org; Newsletter of the International Society of Genetic Genealogy, January 2010. www.isogg.org; *Extra*, "Larry David's Surprising DNA Test on *Lopez Tonight*," November 13, 2009. http://extratv.warnerbros.com.

Four Pharmacogenomic Tests

Pharmacogenomics has emerged as a major component of personalized medicine. The science involves testing people's genes to see how well they react to certain medications. Most pharmacogenomic tests look for gene mutations that help the body break down medications and absorb their components.

Name of test	How it works	What it does
Cytochrome P450 (CYP450) Genotyping Test	The test is effective in determining whether the patient carries gene mutations that help the body absorb about 30 medications. Some people's bodies do not break down the components of drugs, allowing the body to absorb them; therefore, the components remain in the body and may reach high levels that result in dangerous side effects. The test can also tell if the patient carries gene mutations that break down the medications too quickly before they have a chance to work.	The CYP450 test is used to determine the effectiveness of warfarin in stroke and heart attack patients.
Thiopurine Methyltransferase (TPMT) Test	A chemical found in cells known as thiopurine methyltransferase (TPMT) breaks down thiopurine, a drug used to treat leukemia and similar cancers. Some people have genetic variations that prevent them from producing the chemical. As a result, the drug's levels build up in the body, leading to severe side effects.	The TPMT test can check for the genetic variations before treatment begins.
UGT1A1 TA Repeat Genotype Test	The UGT1A1 test detects a variation in a gene that affects how the body breaks down Camptosar, a drug used to treat colorectal cancer. Without the genetic mutation, the medication can reach toxic levels and infect the bone marrow, the spongy interior of bones where new cells are formed. Infection of the bone marrow can be fatal.	Doctors can test for the genetic variation before treatment starts and then customize the dosage to prevent a toxic buildup of the drug.
Dihydropyrimidine Dehydrogenase Test	The test determines how well a chemical found in cells known as dihydropyrimidine dehydrogenase reacts to the anticancer medication 5-fluorouracil (5-FU). Some patients have a genetic variation that results in a decrease in dihydropyrimidine dehydrogenase, which prevents their bodies from absorbing 5-FU. As a result of this deficiency, patients may develop severe or even fatal reactions to 5-FU.	By knowing whether patients have the gene mutation, doctors can tailor doses of 5-FU.

Source: Mayo Clinic, "Pharmacogenomics: When Drug Treatment Becomes Personalized Medicine," June 27, 2008. www.mayoclinic.com.

Key People and Advocacy Groups

American Civil Liberties Union (ACLU): The ACLU has represented clients in cases involving genetic discrimination, privacy issues, racial profiling, and other matters related to genetic testing.

Carrie Buck: The mentally retarded woman was sterilized against her will after the U.S. Supreme Court upheld a Virginia law that enabled mental institutions to sterilize mentally handicapped individuals. Following the 1927 Court ruling, some 60,000 individuals were sterilized in the United States before the practice ended following World War II.

Francis S. Collins: As director of the National Human Genome Research Institute, Collins headed the government team that mapped the human genome, completing the project in 2003. The project has enhanced knowledge of the functions of genes and has laid the groundwork for testing for hundreds of inherited diseases and disorders.

Francis Crick and James D. Watson: The two British biologists discovered the structure of DNA, determining that it is a complicated molecule in the shape of a twisted ladder (the double helix). The work by Crick and Watson laid the groundwork for discoveries of how DNA chemicals fit together, often forming variations known as single nucleotide polymorphisms. These variations help determine a patient's predisposition to develop diseases and disabilities.

Eddy Curry: The American professional basketball player refused to take a genetic test after exhibiting symptoms of an irregular heartbeat. Curry contended that his team had no right to deny him a lucrative contract because it suspected he may be the carrier of a faulty gene. Curry's case set a precedent for the rights of patients in the fight against genetic discrimination.

Greg Fairchild and Tierney Fairchild: An amniocentesis determined the Virginia couple's child would be born with Down syndrome. The Fairchilds wrestled with the decision to terminate the pregnancy and ultimately decided to give birth to the baby girl, whom they named Naia. Their story was told in the 2002 book *Choosing Naia: A Family's Journey*.

Francis Galton: Galton, who first proposed the notion of eugenics, which won widespread support well into the twentieth century, suggested that intelligent people and high achievers limit their marriages to others of similar abilities so they would produce genetically superior offspring. In time, Galton believed, eugenics would result in an overall improvement of the human race.

Robert Guthrie: The microbiologist suspected that phenylketonuria, a condition that causes mental retardation, may be genetically based. To prevent the disease, he recommended that newborns be given blood tests and that if they test high in the amino acid phenylalanine, they should consume diets low in phenylalanine content. An overabundance of phenylalanine causes mental impairment.

Dean Hamer: The genetics researcher at the National Cancer Institute announced in 1993 that he had discovered areas of similarity in the chromosomes of several pairs of gay brothers, suggesting the existence of a "gay gene." Other scientists disputed Hamer's findings, contending that his study group was not broad enough and that the same chromosomal pattern might also be found in heterosexuals.

Mark Hughes: The physician helped pioneer preimplantation genetic diagnosis, which can tell whether embryos created through in vitro fertilization carry genetic mutations that can cause disease. Since helping to develop the science, Hughes has become an advocate against using it to select the gender of children.

Chronology

1859
Charles Darwin suggests that some diseases and debilitations are inherited from parents and other family members.

1953
Francis Crick and James D. Watson discover the structure of the DNA molecule.

1972
Widespread genetic testing commences for sickle-cell anemia; militant black leaders suspect ulterior motives for the tests and urge inner-city blacks to undergo nongenetic testing for the disease.

1927
The U.S. Supreme Court authorizes the involuntary sterilization of Carrie Buck, a mentally retarded woman. The Court's ruling establishes eugenics as a legally permissible policy.

1850   **1930**   **1955**   **1980**

1869
Francis Galton publishes the book *Hereditary Genius*, in which he contends that the human race can be improved if intelligent people limit themselves to marrying others of similar intellects.

1961
Microbiologist Robert Guthrie develops a nongenetic blood test to screen for phenylketonuria, an inherited condition that causes mental retardation.

1945
Following the end of World War II, eugenics falls out of favor after the nature of Nazi genetic experiments are brought to light.

1970
A national program is launched to test Jews of European descent for Tay-Sachs disease.

1974
The Virginia law that permitted the involuntary sterilization of Carrie Buck and others is repealed.

2010
Pathway Genomics agrees to suspend sales of nonprescription direct-to-consumer genetic tests that cost as little as $20 after the FDA says it wants to determine whether such tests should be regulated as medical devices.

1995
Mutations in the BRCA1 and BRCA2 genes are discovered, revealing the causes of most genetically caused breast and ovarian cancer cases.

2003
Separate private and public projects complete their maps of the human genome, identifying all 23,000 genes in the human body.

1984
Law enforcement agencies start matching suspects to crime scenes by comparing their DNA with evidence found at the scenes.

1980   1990   2000   2010

1993
Dean Hamer finds similarities on male chromosomes that he suggests point to the existence of a "gay gene."

2007
Genetic screening reveals that half of all people of European descent carry a gene mutation that increases their risk of heart disease.

1998
Congress authorizes the FBI to establish the Combined DNA Index System, a database of DNA collected from millions of convicted criminals and suspects in crimes.

2008
Congress passes the Genetic Information Nondiscrimination Act, prohibiting insurance companies and employers from using genetic information as a basis for discrimination.

Related Organizations

American Medical Association (AMA)

515 N. State St.

Chicago, IL 60610

phone: (800) 621-8335

Web site: www.ama-assn.org

The national association representing American physicians supports genetic testing and has made many resources about the science available on its Web site. Students can find information about predictive testing of individuals, prenatal testing, and using genetic testing to develop new drug therapies.

Center for Genetics and Society

1936 University Ave., Suite 350

Berkeley, CA 94704

phone: (510) 625-0819 • fax: (510) 625-0874

e-mail: info@geneticsandsociety.org

Web site: www.geneticsandsociety.org

The center is a nonprofit organization that promotes genetic science. The center has posted many resources on its Web site about the impact of genetic testing on society, including essays on eugenics, the creation of DNA databases, and abortion.

Centers for Disease Control and Prevention (CDC)

1600 Clifton Rd. NE

Atlanta, GA 30333

phone: (800) 311-3435

e-mail: cdcinfo@cdc.gov • Web site: www.cdc.gov

The federal government's chief public health agency explores trends in diseases and other conditions that affect the health of Americans. The CDC Web site offers many resources about genetic testing, including government policies that regulate the tests and information on specific diseases that can be detected through genetic screening.

Cystic Fibrosis Foundation

6931 Arlington Rd.

Bethesda, MD 20814

phone: (800) 344-4823 • fax: (301) 951-6378

e-mail: info@cff.org • Web site: www.cff.org

The Cystic Fibrosis Foundation raises money to fund research into cystic fibrosis, a debilitating disease that is caused by a mutated gene. Visitors to the foundation's Web site can find information on carrier and new-born screening for the disease.

Federal Bureau of Investigation (FBI)

J. Edgar Hoover Building

935 Pennsylvania Ave. NW

Washington, DC 20535-0001

phone: (202) 324-3000

Web site: www.fbi.gov

The FBI operates the Combined DNA Index System (CODIS), which contains DNA profiles of nearly 8 million criminal offenders. Visitors to the FBI's Web site can read a background of CODIS and find statistics on the number and types of cases it has helped to solve.

Huntington's Disease Society of America (HDSA)

505 Eighth Ave., Suite 902

New York, NY 10018

phone: (212) 242-1968 • fax: (212) 239-3430

e-mail: hdsainfo@hdsa.org • Web site: www.hdsa.org

The HDSA supports research for a cure for Huntington's disease, which is caused by mutated genes. Students can find a history of the disease on the organization's Web site as well as updates on the latest advancements in the search for a cure.

National Down Syndrome Society (NDSS)

666 Broadway, 8th Floor

New York, NY 10012

phone: (212) 763-4369 • fax: (212) 979-2873

e-mail: info@ndss.org • Web site: www.ndss.org

The NDSS promotes research and education about the disorder, which is caused by a chromosomal imbalance and is detectable through prenatal genetic testing. Visitors to the organization's Web site can find information on the history and causes of the disorder as well as statistics on the number of Americans born with Down syndrome.

National Human Genome Research Institute

National Institutes of Health

Building 31, Room 4B09

31 Center Dr., MSC 2152

9000 Rockville Pike

Bethesda, MD 20892-2152

phone: (301) 402-0911 • fax: (301) 402-2218

Web site: www.genome.gov

The National Human Genome Research Institute headed the federal government's project to map the human genome. Visitors to the agency's Web site can read an overview of the project and how the genome is assisting in the development of genetic tests. The Web site also includes an archive of information on the discovery and characteristics of DNA.

National Institutes of Health (NIH)

9000 Rockville Pike

Bethesda, MD 20892

phone: (301) 496-4000

e-mail: nihinfo@od.nih.gov • Web site: www.nih.gov

The NIH is the chief funding arm of the federal government for medical research. Many resources about genetic testing are available on the agency's

Web site, where students can download a copy of the NIH publication *Genetic Testing: What It Means for Your Health and Your Family's Health.*

U.S. Food and Drug Administration (FDA)

5600 Fishers Ln.

Rockville, MD 20857-0001

phone: (888) 463-6332

Web site: www.fda.gov

The FDA approves all drug therapies available to Americans, including those that fall under the science of personalized medicine. Visitors to the FDA's Web site can find background on personalized medicine, which is under the authority of the agency's Division of Personalized Nutrition and Medicine.

For Further Research

Books

Ruth Schwartz Cowan, *Heredity and Hope: The Case for Genetic Screening*. Cambridge, MA: Harvard University Press, 2008.

Masha Gessen, *Blood Matters: From Inherited Illness to Designer Babies, How the World and I Found Ourselves in the Future of the Gene*. New York: Harcourt, 2008.

Ronald M. Green, *Babies by Design: The Ethics of Genetic Choice*. New Haven, CT: Yale University Press, 2008.

Joi L. Morris and Ora K. Gordon, *Positive Results: Making the Best Decisions When You're at High Risk for Breast or Ovarian Cancer*. New York: Prometheus, 2010.

Philip R. Reilly, *The Strongest Boy in the World: How Genetic Information Is Reshaping Our Lives*. Cold Spring Harbor, NY: Cold Spring Harbor Laboratory, 2010.

Jan A. Witkowski and John R. Inglis, eds., *Davenport's Dream: 21st Century Reflections on Heredity and Eugenics*. Cold Spring Harbor, NY: Cold Spring Harbor Laboratory, 2008.

Doris Teichler Zallen, *To Test or Not to Test*. New Brunswick, NJ: Rutgers University Press, 2008.

Periodicals

Anjana Ahuja, "Please, God, Can I Have a Daughter Next?" *Times (London)*, February 4, 2010.

Amy Harmon, "Insurance Fears Lead Many to Shun DNA Tests," *New York Times*, February 24, 2008.

Dominique Jackson, "One Woman's Journey: Taking the Risk of Breast Cancer Seriously," *Seattle Post-Intelligencer*, April 9, 2010.

Julia Langdon and Shelley Thoupos, "Would You Abort a Baby with Down's Syndrome?" *Daily Mail (London)*, October 29, 2009.

Jim Manzi, "Undetermined: There Is Danger in Assuming That Genes Explain All," *National Review*, June 2, 2008.

Solomon Moore, "FBI and States Vastly Expand DNA Databases," *New York Times*, April 19, 2009.

Steven Pinker, "My Genome, Myself," *New York Times*, January 11, 2009.

Andrew Pollack, "Genetic Test May Reveal Source of Mystery Tumors," *New York Times*, March 10, 2009.

Wanda Reed, "Weighing the Benefits of Genetic Testing," *Seattle Woman*, April 2009.

John Ward, "Bush OKs Bill on Genetic Bias," *Washington Times*, May 22, 2008.

Web Sites

Georgetown University National Reference Center for Bioethics Literature: Genetic Testing and Genetic Screening (http://bioethics.george town.edu/publications/scopenotes/sn22.htm#essay). Sponsored by Georgetown University in Washington, D.C., the center examines moral and ethical issues that surface during medical procedures. The center's report on genetic testing examines such issues as privacy, discrimination, and whether teenagers and other young people should undergo genetic testing.

Mayo Clinic: Genetic Testing (www.mayoclinic.com/health/genetic testing/MY00370). The nationally renowned research hospital based in Rochester, Minnesota, provides an overview of genetic testing on its Web site. Visitors can learn about many issues involved in genetic testing, such as the future of pharmacogenomics and prenatal testing, by reading the blog entries of Carrie A. Zabel, the clinic's genetic counselor.

National Cancer Institute, "BRCA1 and BRCA2: Cancer Risk and Genetic Testing" (www.cancer.gov/cancertopics/factsheet/Risk/BRCA). The Web page sponsored by the National Cancer Institute provides extensive information on the BRCA gene mutations that cause breast and ovarian cancers. Visitors can learn how people can be tested for the mutations and how to interpret the test results.

Source Notes

Overview

1. Doris Teichler Zallen, *To Test or Not to Test*. New Brunswick, NJ: Rutgers University Press, 2008, pp. 1–2.
2. Quoted in Kirsten Weir, "Self Help," *Current Science*, February 22, 2008, p. 10.
3. Quoted in Weir, "Self Help."
4. Quoted in Andrew Pollack, "Genetic Test May Reveal Source of Mystery Tumors," *New York Times*, March 10, 2009, p. 6.
5. Quoted in Deborah Franklin, "Family Struggles with Ambiguity of Genetic Testing," National Public Radio, December 30, 2008. www.npr.org.
6. United States Conference of Catholic Bishops, "The Promise and Peril of Genetic Screening," March 1996. www.usccb.org.
7. Zallen, *To Test or Not to Test*, p. 127.
8. Quoted in Mike McGraw, "Things Getting Testy: Curry's Attorney Won't Agree to Bulls' Demand," *Arlington Heights (IL) Daily Herald*, September 24, 2005, p. 1.
9. Quoted in Jim Litke, "Curry's DNA Fight with Bulls 'Bigger than Sports World,'" ESPN, September 28, 2005. http://sports.espn.go.com.
10. Doris Teichler Zallen, *Does It Run in the Family? A Consumer's Guide to DNA Testing for Genetic Disorders*. New Brunswick, NJ: Rutgers University Press, 1997, p. 148.
11. Quoted in Claudia Kalb, Barbie Nadeau, and Sarah Schafer, "Brave New Babies," *Newsweek*, February 2, 2004. www.newsweek.com.

How Beneficial Is Genetic Testing for Diseases?

12. Quoted in Jerome Groopman, "Decoding Destiny," *New Yorker*, February 9, 1998, p. 42.
13. Hereditary Disease Foundation, "Guidelines for Genetic Testing for Huntington's Disease," 1994. www.hdfoundation.org.
14. Quoted in Associated Press, "Stomachs Removed on Basis of Genetic Tests," *USA Today*, June 20, 2001. www.usatoday.com.
15. Zallen, *To Test or Not to Test*, pp. 40–41.
16. National Cancer Institute, "BRCA1 and BRCA2: Cancer Risk and Genetic Testing," March 29, 2009. www.cancer.gov.
17. Zallen, *To Test or Not to Test*, p. 87.
18. Quoted in Wanda Reed, "Weighing the Benefits of Genetic Testing," *Seattle Woman*, April 2009. www.seattlewomanmagazine.com.
19. Quoted in Jennifer Goodwin, "Newer Genetic Test for Autism More Effective," *BusinessWeek*, March 15, 2010. www.businessweek.com.
20. Quoted in Jennifer Couzin and Jocelyn Kaiser, "Closing the Net on Common Disease Genes," *Science*, May 11, 2007, p. 822.
21. Zallen, *To Test or Not to Test*, p. 3.

How Does Genetic Testing Influence Family Planning?

22. Quoted in Mitchell Zuckoff, *Choosing Naia: A Family's Journey*. Boston: Beacon, 2002, p. 120.
23. Quoted in Jill Lepore, "Fixed," *New Yorker*, March 29, 2010, p. 95.
24. Ruth Schwartz Cowan, *Heredity and Hope: The Case for Genetic Screening*. Cambridge, MA: Harvard University Press, 2008, p. 112.
25. William McKeever, "Abortion and LDS Inconsistency," Mormonism Research Ministry, April 8, 2002. www.mrm.org.
26. Julia Langdon and Shelley Thoupos, "Would You Abort a Baby with Down's Syndrome?" *Daily Mail (London)*, October 28, 2009, p. 20.

27. Quoted in Sarah Nightingale, "Syndrome Study: Researchers Hope to Help Down Syndrome Families," *Lubbock (TX) Avalanche-Journal*, January 25, 2010. www.lubbockonline.com.

28. Quoted in Nightingale, "Syndrome Study."

29. Cowan, *Heredity and Hope*, p. 143.

30. Quoted in Sue MacDonald, "Sickle Cell Testing Stirs Ethical Debate," *Cincinnati Enquirer*, September 15, 1999. www.enquirer.com.

31. Ronald M. Green, "Building Baby from the Genes Up," *Washington Post*, April 13, 2008. www.washingtonpost.com.

Will Genetic Testing Lead to Discrimination?

32. Quoted in Cowan, *Heredity and Hope*, p. 177.

33. Richard Horton, "Is Homosexuality Inherited?" *New York Review of Books*, July 1995. www.nybooks.com.

34. Quoted in Traci Watson and Joseph P. Shapiro, "Is There a 'Gay Gene?'" *U.S. News & World Report*, November 13, 1995, p. 93.

35. Quoted in Amy Harmon, "Insurance Fears Lead Many to Shun DNA Tests," *New York Times*, February 24, 2008. www.nytimes.com.

36. Quoted in Harmon, "Insurance Fears Lead Many to Shun DNA Tests."

37. Quoted in John Ward, "Bush OKs Bill on Genetic Bias," *Washington Times*, May 22, 2008, p. A-4.

38. Zallen, *To Test or Not to Test*, p. 140.

39. Quoted in Richard Willing, "White House Seeks to Expand DNA Database," *USA Today*, April 15, 2003. www.usatoday.com.

40. Quoted in Willing, "White House Seeks to Expand DNA Database."

41. Quoted in Solomon Moore, "FBI and States Vastly Expand DNA Databases," *New York Times*, April 19, 2009, p. A-1.

42. Quoted in Richard Willing, "DNA Offers Clues to Suspect's Race," *USA Today*, August 16, 2005. www.usatoday.com.

43. Elizabeth Cohen, "The Government Has Your Baby's DNA," CNN, February 4, 2010. www.cnn.com.

What Is the Future of Genetic Testing?

44. Quoted in Liz Szabo, "New Cancer Treatments Are Coming Made to Order," *USA Today*, June 3, 2004, p. 9-D.

45. Quoted in Bruce R. Posten, "Personalized Treatment Comes to the Forefront," *Reading (PA) Eagle*, October 13, 2009. http://readingeagle.com.

46. Quoted in Michelle Meadows, "Genomics and Personalized Medicine," *FDA Consumer*, November/December 2005, p. 12.

47. Quoted in Audrey Grayson, "Gene Test Can Indicate Whether Tamoxifen Can Fight Breast Cancer," ABC News, December, 17, 2007. http://abcnews.go.com.

48. Quoted in Graeme Smith, "DNA Testing 'Is Potentially Inaccurate and Harmful,'" *Glasgow Herald*, September 25, 2008, p. 11.

49. Quoted in Rita Rubin, "A 'Wild West' Way of Telling Baby's Sex?" *USA Today*, July 16, 2007, p. 6-D.

50. Quoted in Rubin, "A 'Wild West' Way of Telling Baby's Sex?"

51. Quoted in Rebecca Leung, "Choose the Sex of Your Baby: New Technology May Allow Couples to Design the Perfect Baby," CBS News, August 11, 2004. www.cbsnews.com.

52. Quoted in Leung, "Choose the Sex of Your Baby."

53. Quoted in Claudia Kalb, "In Our Blood: DNA Testing—It Is Connecting Lost Cousins and Giving Families Surprising Glimpses into Their Pasts," *Newsweek*, February 6, 2006, p. 46.

54. Quoted in Hsien-Hsien Lei, "Eye on DNA Interview: Dr. Tzung-Fu Hsieh of Red Tracer DNA Test for the Red Hair Gene, MC1R," Eye on DNA, January 26, 2009. www.eyeondna.com.

List of Illustrations

List of Illustrations

Index

About the Author

Hal Marcovitz, a writer based in Chalfont, Pennsylvania, has written more than 150 books for young readers. His other titles in the Compact Research series include *Asthma*, *Painkillers*, *Religious Fundamentalism*, *Bipolar Disorder*, *Phobias*, *Hepatitis*, and *Meningitis*.